Sailor Jerry's
Tattoo Stencils

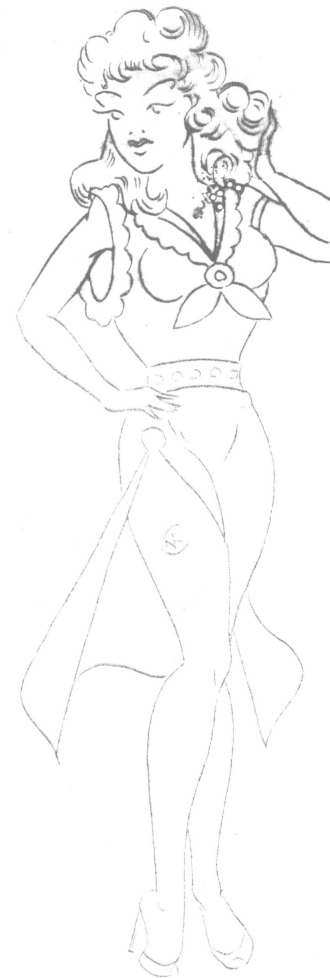

Kate Hellenbrand

with Foreword by Matty Jankowski

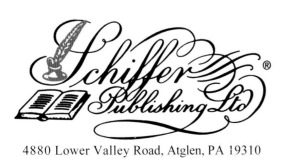

Schiffer Publishing Ltd®

4880 Lower Valley Road, Atglen, PA 19310

On the cover: The tools of the trade are seen in this recreated scene from Sailor Jerry's art table during a typical stencil cutting session. First, the designs were drawn and painted with watercolors on heavy paper. These sheets of brilliant designs were called "flash" (a carnival term referring to flash placards that were designed to quickly grab the attention of a wandering crowd). Almost always, stencils would be cut at the same time that a flash sheet was finished, eliminating the need to cut stencils later. Time was often of the essence and as soon as a sheet of flash was ready to display, the stencils needed to be ready for immediate placement on the body.

Seen here are flash sheets and blank sheets of acetate. A pinvise was used to hold a standard 78 rpm vinyl record needle. This was the etching tool, held like a pencil. The tattoo artist would place a sheet of soft acetate or celluloid over the design to be traced and any foundation line pertinent for the successful duplication of the design would be cut into the plastic. When the stencil was finished, a sprinkling of black graphite powder (from a standard salt shaker) would be rubbed into all the carved grooves. The stencil would then be pressed against the client's prepared skin (recently shaved and moisturized with a thin film of petroleum jelly). The carbon in the stencil's grooves would adhere to the skin's slightly sticky surface. When the stencil was pulled away, the carbon would (hopefully) stick to the skin, leaving a thin, fragile outline to be followed by the tattoo machine. Artists nearly always signed their flash on the front and back of the sheet. They also often signed the corresponding stencils.

The elements on the cover of this book are all original Sailor Jerry artifacts and were used by him in the creation of his acetate stencils. All items seen here are from the author's collection.

Back cover: Kate Hellenbrand at work. Photo: Greg Mango

Pages 1-16 designed by Bonnie M. Hensley
Pages 17-96 designed by Kate Hellenbrand
Cover designed by Bruce M. Waters with an image stylized by the author
Type set in Rage Italic/Korinna BT

ISBN: 978-0-7643-1562-6
Printed in China

Schiffer Books are available at special discounts for bulk purchases for sales promotions or premiums. Special editions, including personalized covers, corporate imprints, and excerpts can be created in large quantities for special needs. For more information contact the publisher:

Published by Schiffer Publishing Ltd.
4880 Lower Valley Road
Atglen, PA 19310
Phone: (610) 593-1777; Fax: (610) 593-2002
E-mail: Info@schifferbooks.com

For the largest selection of fine reference books on this and related subjects, please visit our website at
www.schifferbooks.com
We are always looking for people to write books on new and related subjects. If you have an idea for a book please contact us at the above address.

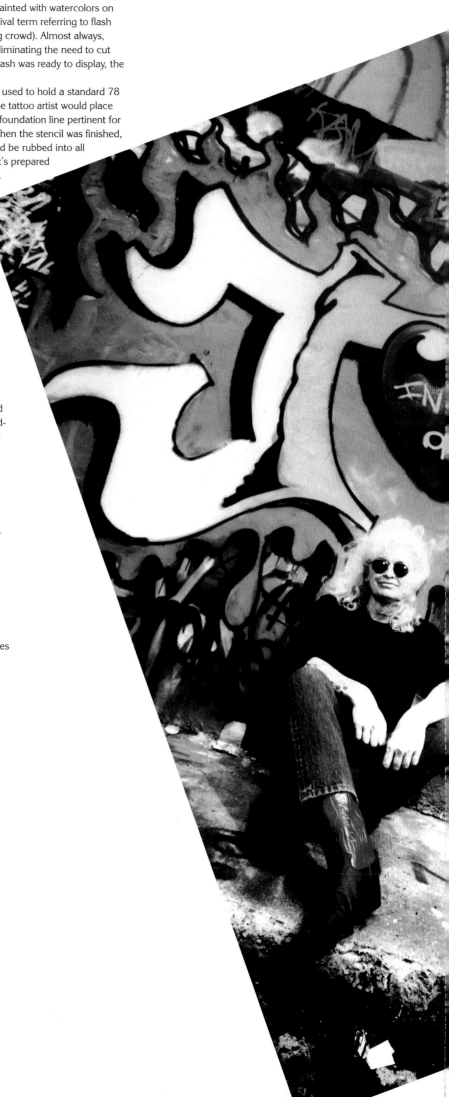

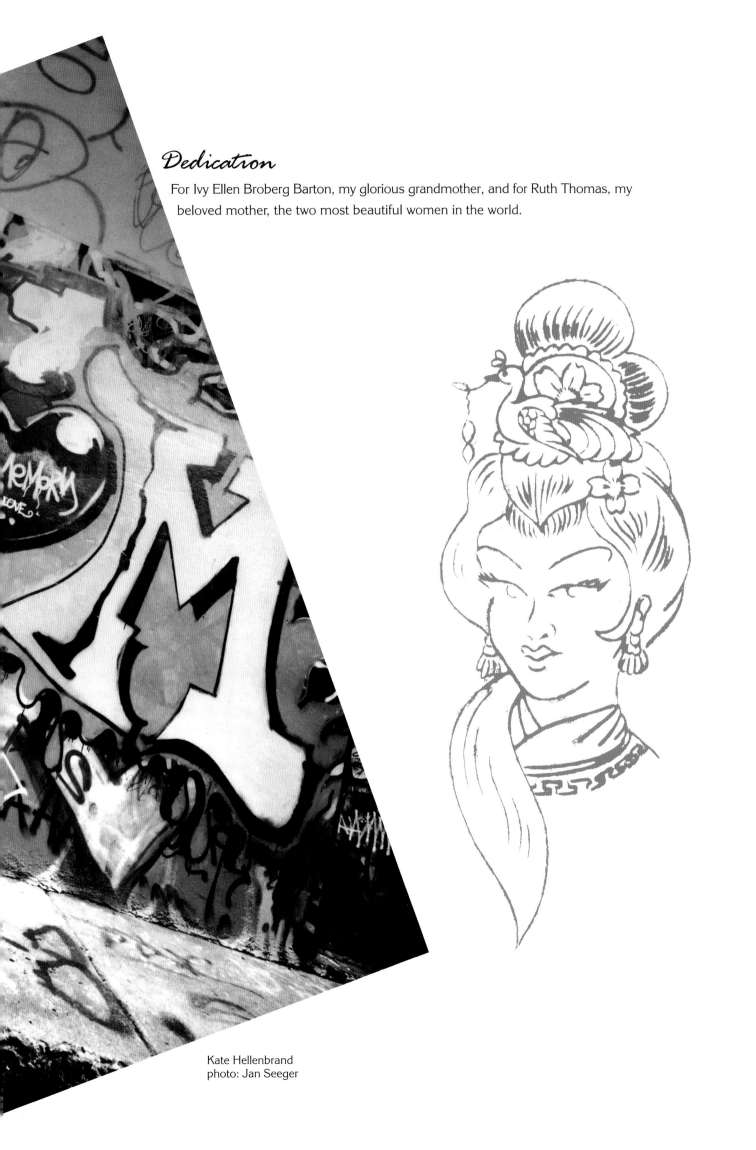

Dedication

For Ivy Ellen Broberg Barton, my glorious grandmother, and for Ruth Thomas, my beloved mother, the two most beautiful women in the world.

Kate Hellenbrand
photo: Jan Seeger

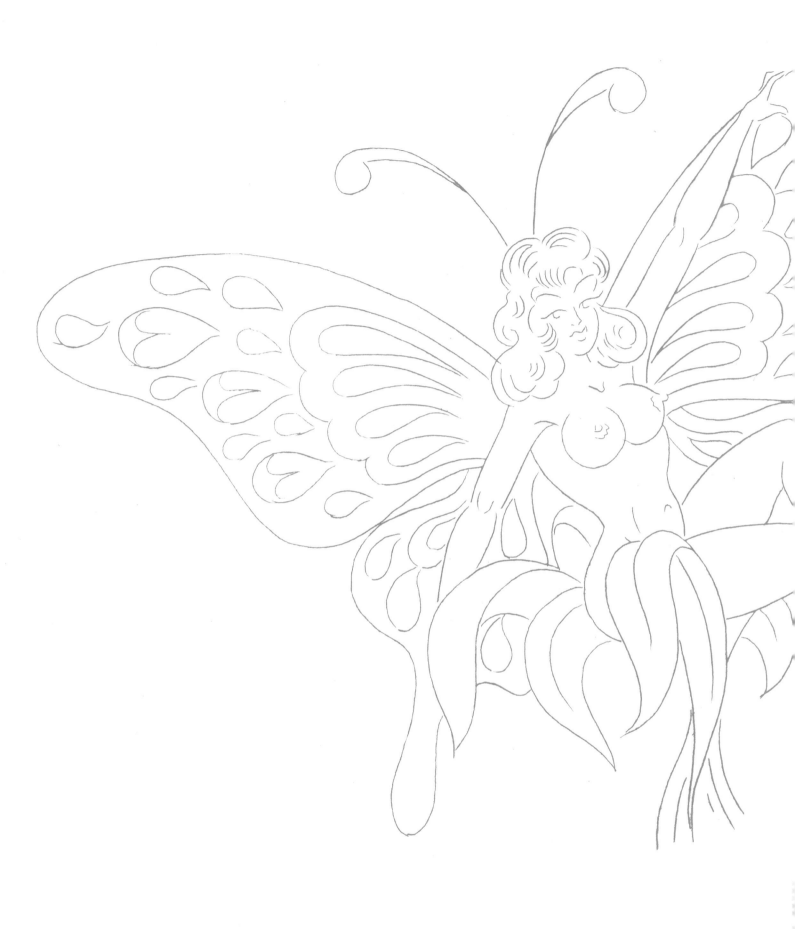

Contents

Acknowledgments

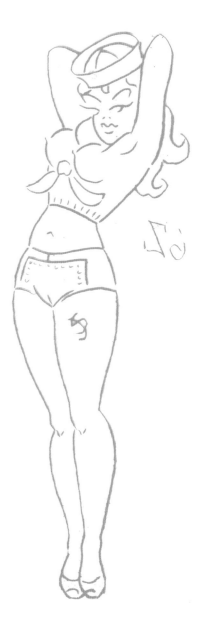

It is trite but true; I owe a debt to everyone I've ever met for their life's lessons.

My profound thanks goes to those closest to me in New York City who allow me to do what I love to do with the greatest support: Wes Wood; Matty Jankowski; Danielle DiStefano; Crag, Anna and Cain; my fellow artists at Sacred Tattoo; the floor personnel who work behind the scenes with little recognition.

I thank my new friends at Schiffer Publishing: Peter, Joe, Tina and all the smiling voices at the end of the phones.

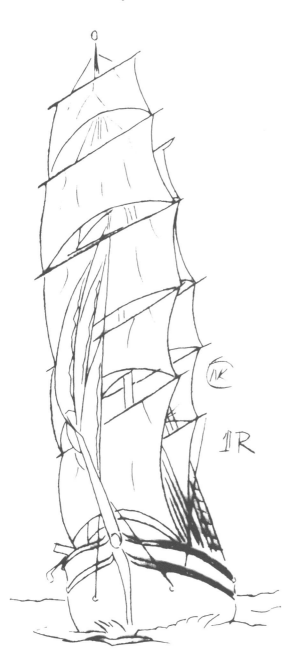

Special thanks to tattoo artist Mike Wilson of Florida for my new Mom tattoo seen here and to photographer Bill DeMichele for documenting this important event.

My most special thanks go to those who have listened and loved me all these years: Jane, Joan, Jan, Merrily, Corky, Julie, Kerri, and Allison.

Of course I thank my family who have supported me even when they didn't understand: Uncle Dale, Waldo, Margaret, and Uncle Jack.

My gratitude goes to everyone in the tattoo community, especially the old-schoolers, but also the new kids on the block. Thanks to Bill Funk, Mario Barth, Trevor Marshall, Don and Flo at National Tattoo Association, and Lou Robbins. I especially thank those who were there in the beginning for setting the standard of excellence. I was privileged to know Zeke Owens, Don Ed Hardy, Jack Rudy, Thom DeVita, Bob Roberts; Jamie "La Palma" Summers, Paul Rogers, and most specifically, Norman Keith "Sailor Jerry" Collins.

Foreword

Matty Jankowski

Body art, spanning centuries and cultures, includes many varied methods of application. The ancient art of tattoo and its rites, rituals, and decoration, have been transformed into a modern American folk art. Twentieth century icons of Americana have a significant place in tattoo history, but none greater than those of Sailor Jerry Collins, an artist often imitated from Hamburg to Hong Kong and New Zealand to New York. His full color designs and their conversion into stencils used to transform these designs from lines on paper to indelible marks on skin comprised a skilled craft much like tattooing. Preserved as a permanent record, each tattoo had a corresponding mirror image etched in acetate or celluloid using a stylus or pin vise. The yellowed, cloudy and spattered, charcoal-encrusted stencils were used time and again to transfer the outline patterns.

Certain rites, rituals, and marks of identity have endured through sailors, soldiers, and service men and women worldwide. Western culture is devoid of rites of passage and, consciously or unconsciously, tattoos are worn for protection, empowerment, commemoration, memorial, or identification with a specific group or belief. Being tattooed is about fear and transformation, decoration, or just plain fun.

These one-of-a-kind artifacts are sold at galleries, exhibited at museums, and prized by collectors worldwide. They have been preserved from the past by tattooist Kate Hellenbrand. There is a wide range of designs, from rituals of the sea, with bluebirds, pigs, roosters, and hinges to mermaids, pirate girl pinups, hula honeys, classic hearts, horse shoes, roses, daggers, butterflies, bunnies, skunks, donkeys, and more than a barrel full of monkeys.

Both traditional designs and Jerry's quest to push the limits by creating exotic elaborate tattoos in his recognizable style are evident in this magnificent collection.

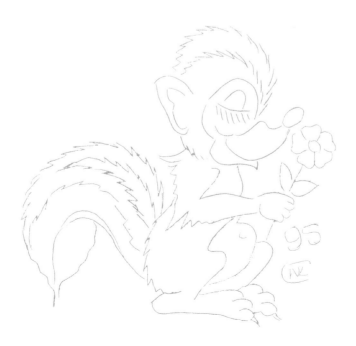

Preface

In 1971 I was living in New York City working full time as a graphic designer and typographer at a leading advertising agency on Fifth Avenue and 53rd Street. One of my clients was the nearby Museum of American Folk Art.

At night, I was also developing a friendship of sorts with several local New York collectors and "underground" tattoo artists. (Tattooing had been banned for nearly a decade by the New York City government, lending an even greater aura of intrigue to this already mysterious folk art.)

When I learned that the Museum of American Folk Art was interested in mounting an exhibit on tattooing, it seemed natural to approach curators there with the prospect of incorporating a contemporary section to their historical presentation. The idea was accepted and I found myself fully immersed in the tattoo world. My participation in the show was to help seek out notable international tattoo artists, solicit biographies, drawings, photographs, and anecdotal information for exhibit. My search lead to several American tattoo artists: Ed Hardy, Zeke Owens, Don Nolan, and Cliff Raven. They, unanimously, pointed me in the direction of Sailor Jerry Collins of Honolulu, Hawaii.

After the exhibit ended, I continued my friendships with many of the participating artists. I had, by this time, started to tattoo — the great gift of living canvas first offered to me by Tom King of the Bronx. For his part, I believe he wanted free tattoos. I was interested in learning how the tools worked.

With little guidance, I etched first a small flower on Tom's lower leg, then a large peacock in the middle of his chest. Later, I "sleeved" his right arm by filling in every bit of available space not already occupied by other tattoos. My design was a dragon climbing through clouds, running from Tom's wrist to his shoulder. I was so enraptured by the time-space elasticity of tattooing and its immediacy that I soon quit my graphics job and became a full-time tattoo artist.

Destiny intervened in 1972 when I was invited to be one of seven artists at what was to be the first international tattoo convention in Hawaii, hosted by Sailor Jerry Collins. He dubbed us "The Council of the Seven."

The Council lasted approximately a week. When the other attendees left, I remained behind with Jerry to work for another several weeks. Although I had only begun my tattoo career, Jerry opened his home and shop to me, requiring that I work from 3 p.m. to closing (usually around 10:00 p.m.), just as he'd demand of a regular, (i.e. male) apprentice.

Sailor Jerry disliked the many newcomers in the business and he was even less tolerant of women of any age coming into it. Yet, when I arrived at his door for this landmark Council, I was welcomed wholeheartedly.

I learned many things from Jerry during this short time but nothing more important than how a tattoo artist should think about the art and their place in it. Jerry was notorious at fending off disrespectful or irritating customers. He was a master at shop talk, whether he was dealing with a drunk marine or a shy college coed. He was an imposing man with little tolerance for fakery and falseness. He suffered no fools.

Jerry was intelligent and street smart. He could curse like the sailor he was or he could seduce like a Shakespearian actor, his mellifluous voice rolling like distant thunder. He was happy living an isolated life in Hawaii where his primary clientele was the young military personnel stationed there. He was a prolific tattoo artist, working nonstop during military paydays in his tiny downtown Honolulu shop. When the military business slowed down between paydays, Jerry worked on the locals, concentrating on the young women of the Islands.

Jerry had demanding and diverse interests which he invariably pursued to the professional level. He played saxophone with his own dance band, he piloted boatloads of tourists around Waikiki as the only licensed skipper of a huge, three-masted schooner moored in Honolulu harbor. He had a late-night radio talk show wherein he lectured against the impending (as he saw it) downfall of the American political system by infiltration of liberals. He was a prolific writer and carried on in-depth communications with many pen-pals throughout the world.

At the shop, he was constantly innovating. He found better power sources, manufactured new machine frame configurations, and invented needle setups. He sought out and found color pigments that were nontoxic and safe. To ensure their safety he would tattoo these discoveries into his lower legs. If the colors reacted, he'd dig them out and try the next batch.

When a tooth gave him trouble, he took a hammer and chopstick and knocked out the offender with a solid whack. He cured his own skin cancer by tattooing prescription medicines meant to be taken internally directly onto the malignant areas.

Jerry was a consummate practical joker of incomparable magnitude. Often the entire city of Honolulu would have to halt "business as usual" because of one of his pranks. One favorite was the time he strapped a giant salami and two hairy coconuts just below the golden belt on the revered statue of King Kamehameha, right before the beginning of the King Kamehameha Day parade. Floats, marching bands, majorettes, and dignitaries had to stand in the hot Hawaiian sun until workers could find a ladder large enough to scramble up to and cut down the offending pornographic appendages. He was never found out for his many elaborate escapades.

I cleaned the shop, set up his station before his next project. I checked the points of his needles, filled and emptied the autoclave, and bagged and stored the equipment in his desiccator.

I listened. I watched. I bantered with customers, sitting in the sultry tropical shop, the air carrying the fragrance of teriyaki sauce, the customers smelling like coconuts. I did what an "old-school" apprentice did. His teaching was covert. If I couldn't devise what he was doing by watching, I would have to hint and wait for the answer. Ours was a verbal dance. Had I appeared any more eager, the flow of information would have stopped immediately. Asking any overt question was forbidden.

My gender was a source of constant flirtation on his part. Whenever a young woman came into the shop, Jerry would look over at me and wink. And then he would begin to do what no other tattoo artist had yet accomplished — he'd do single-needle, tiny, highly detailed, full color designs on her hip or abdominal area. He wasn't concerned that he was inventing a style of tattooing, which he dubbed "Feminigraphics." He was more excited that he could, at his age, still look at young women, embellish their bodies and possibly get a snapshot afterwards for his photo albums. "I've never had it so good," he wrote, describing his latest project in a letter to me in 1973. "These pretty young girls are going to make a dirty old man out of me yet."

His letters to me were disclosures of matters of his heart, disappointments, emotional attachments, interspersed with technical data and gossip about the tattoo scene in Hawaii.

I was the least likely candidate for this kind of relationship with him. I represented the two things he disliked the most in tattooers: youthful inexperience and being female. However, his real nature overrode his prejudices. His gifts to me were of generosity, patience, friendship, and understanding. He was a teacher, a role model, a rascal, an innovator, and a legend.

When Sailor Jerry died in 1973, I was living in San Diego. After I got the phone call, I drove to the beach and watched the Pacific Ocean roll in and out at my feet. Hours later, I went home, called my Grandmother and borrowed the money to make a down payment on his estate.

In the past 30 years, I have cared for and watched over my collection of his stencils. I have always been able to turn to them — these "tattoos in plastic" — for comfort. They are magical vectors for my memories. They are indescribably beautiful to me. They hold Jerry's energy, his life's force, frozen in time. I offer them now to those who revere his contributions and his influence. These are critically important. They helped him do the impossible: make the world a more beautiful place, one person at a time.

Chapter One: *The Acetate Tattoo Stencil*

We are experiencing an unprecedented global explosion in body modification. Tattooing and piercing have become the fastest growing businesses today. One pragmatic reason for this rapid growth comes from a practical source: the ease of applying a design's basic line work to the skin. The introduction of the indelible thermo-copier stencil has replaced the difficult and problematic acetate stencil, enabling novice tattooists to bypass what was once the most difficult parts of tattooing — the fragile, unstable graphite stencil imprint.

How does a drawing get transferred from the wall to the client's skin? Since the dawn of time, tattooists had to "draw" designs on their client's skin. As tattoos became increasingly popular around the turn of the 20th century, however, the burgeoning economic factor became apparent and custom drawing became time-consuming and tedious (not to mention often inaccurate).

New York City Bowery-area tattooist Stanley Moskowitz relates how his father, Willie, began to look for another more efficient and speedy way to get clients in and out of the chair (and the greenbacks out of their wallets). Stan, his brother, Walter, and Willie began to carve tattoo outlines into plastic (celluloid or acetate) sheets that were soft enough to bend over the client's body. By etching the design's fundamental line work into the plastic and rubbing graphite into the carved grooves, they could use the same stencil over and over, rapidly and almost endlessly.

These indestructible stencils, however, left behind a fragile line of graphite that floated on a thin film of petroleum jelly. This thin line would disappear with the slightest disturbance. If a rotating fan was operating nearby, the imprint could be literally blown away. If a misbehaving machine sputtered or spit, the image could be lost. If an artist inadvertently touched the arm with a tissue, if the client happened to brush his body against a chair or table, the stencil could disappear.

The artist always had to begin working the design from the bottom corner, progressing up into the design. Designs with long lines (pinups, banners, or the outline of an eagle feather) were a nightmare. The artist had to gulp, grip, grin, and bear down.

Acetate stencils required an aggressive approach. There was no turning back once the tattoo was begun. If the stencil lines disappeared, the tattoo artist could only imagine where they had once been and forge ahead. You had to know how to finish the design without the client ever seeing you sweat.

Trying to reapply the stencil over already worked skin was considered bad form. The style of tattooing at the time was rugged and raw. Very often the skin was welted and bleeding. Reapplying a stencil over open skin would not only look incompetent but make a bigger mess. It would also contaminate the stencil. Sometimes the tattooist would revert to the pre-stencil days, drawing the remainder of the design on the skin, usually using a toothpick dipped in the black ink pot.

Once the tattoo was finished, the stencil would be cleaned off with alcohol and put back in a drawer, or on a peg or in an envelope to await the next use.

Cutting the stencils was no easy task. Usually this chore was passed on to the tattooist's apprentice, great training for many a beginner trying to break into the trade.

Holding a pin vise with a 78 rpm phonograph needle as the point, a clean piece of acetate (or celluloid) would be placed over the desired design. The tattooist would then pin down the edges of the acetate so that it couldn't shift during the cutting process.

It was necessary to cut lines that were smooth, precise and evenly deep. Many times the stencil had to be thrown away because the lines were cut too deeply or not deeply enough.

Acetates had another downside. Over time, the acetates would begin to decompose, just as Hollywood is discovering with its older, silent films. Some older stencils also cast off fumes and, with charcoal or graphite still embedded in the grooves, it was not uncommon for a box of stencils to self-ignite, bursting into flames. Several shops have, over the years, burned to the ground because an old box of acetate stencils stored in the attic self-combusted. Acetates also had to be constantly updated and refined. They were a never-ending dilemma.

But Moskowitz insists that acetate stencils still have their place. In 2001, Stanley celebrates 57 years of slinging ink. He still advocates acetates when he needs to cover an old tattoo. "How are you going to see what you're covering and line it up properly if you don't use an acetate stencil?" he asks. Because of the acetate's transparency, it is easy to align a new design over the old.

Acetates held a place of honor for some 50 years in the field of tattooing. But they were unreliable and very difficult to use, requiring patience and perseverance to succeed. Contemporary artists use a pressure/heat sensitive copier to create a gentian-violet style stencil that is nearly indelible, allowing the tattooist to begin working at any point within a tattoo design. Only alcohol will remove the stencil's image from the skin and the artist can work for hours without losing the pattern. "Thermofaxes can make tattooists out of rhesus monkeys," was a favorite theory of the late Sailor Moses of Mississippi.

These newfangled paper stencils are tissue-thin and extremely fragile. They are used only once and thrown away. The stencil collectible will not be a product of this era.

Acetate stencils are beautiful relics, many still encrusted with the graphite of their years in service. They are rich testimonies to the struggle and strength of the mid-century tattoo artist.

While tattoos may be transient in their very nature, vibrant only as long as the patron still lives, these tattoos in plastic can live on for generations.

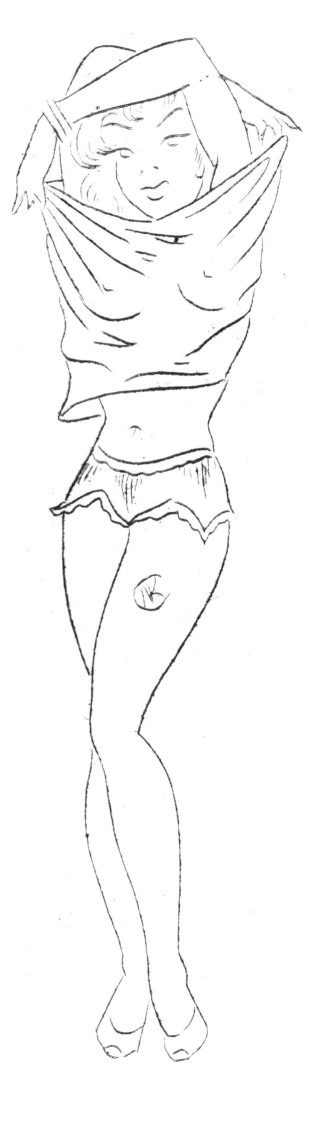

Chapter Two: *Sailor Jerry, Redefining an Ancient Art*

In every area of human endeavor there stands one or two individuals who innovate and reform their chosen field so totally that it is impossible to envision how their worlds could exist if they had not been born.

Norman Keith Collins (also known as Sailor Jerry) was such an innovator, a true renaissance man, transforming the ancient art form of tattooing so completely that it can be divided into two eras — pre- and post-Sailor Jerry. His influence was phenomenal in every aspect of this strange hybrid of art and science, called the oldest art form, pre-dating recorded history.

Sailor Jerry Collins of Honolulu, Hawaii, has been called the American Tattoo Master. His influence on the field of tattooing cannot be measured. From 1936 to his death in 1973, Collins was relentless in his crusade to elevate tattooing in every way possible. There is not one aspect of the art form that Jerry did not revolutionize. His inventions and renovations covered everything from sanitation and health concerns to the discoveries of new pigments. He brought his considerable intellect to bear on the tools of the trade, fine-tuning (if you will) the power packs and machines themselves. He invented new needle configurations that would more easily coax ink into skin without trauma. He also fiercely defended a philosophy that endorsed tattoo artists as latter-day shamans with no apology.

Probably Jerry's most notable contributions were his tattoo designs. Prior to Jerry's plump and sensual style, tattoos had been somewhat primitive, thin and rough. Jerry's vision — strong line composition, ruthless fields of black shading and the introduction of his new color discoveries — allowed everything to blossom under his touch. His strongest legacy, however, would be his cheese-cake pinups. He is the Vargas, the Elvgren, the Frazetta of tattoo pinup designs. He created a bounty of busty, wasp-waisted, long-legged luscious dreamgirls, unequalled before or since.

Jerry's greatest hope was that his beloved world of tattooing would be taken seriously and he sought to set a new, higher standard for the craft.

Until now, only a very small portion of his work has been seen in museums or galleries and his flash found in "Outsider" exhibitions of self-taught folk artists.

This book is the first significant compilation in print of many of Jerry's stencils. The bulk of his images have been controlled by a handful of tattoo/folk art collectors. Finally, one collector is choosing to share her collection of Sailor Jerry's hand-carved acetate and celluloid stencils — the newest "tattoo collectible." They are, in the best sense, permanent tattoos in plastic, hand carved by Sailor Jerry for use in his tattoo shop in Honolulu.

This book is a catalog of Sailor Jerry's stencils. They remain in their original condition and are shown at exact size. Each stencil was signed with one of Jerry's distinctive signatures. The numbers and letters were part of Jerry's filing system.

In most cases only one stencil of each image exists. When two were cut, they would be "right" or "left" stencils, as most designs aesthetically face into the center of the body. Through this catalog, it is possible to witness Jerry's design evolution. (He would update favorite money-making designs — refining the face, the hair, whatever he needed to make the design more contemporary.)

This book offers a singular opportunity to review a master's work, purchase a piece of tattoo history, and perpetuate a timeless art.

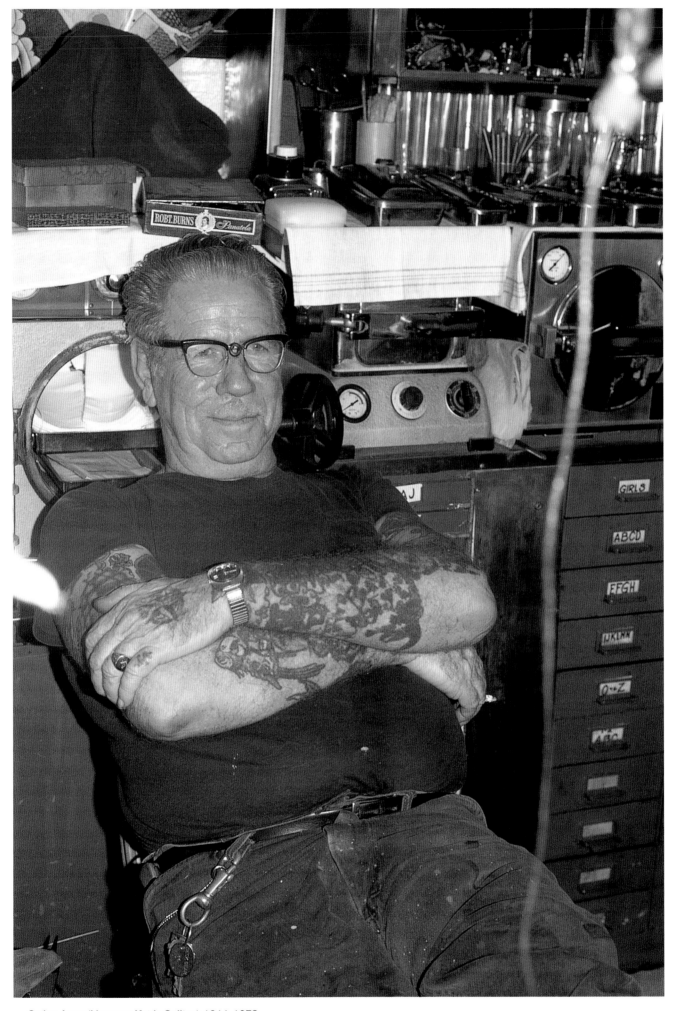

Sailor Jerry (Norman Keith Collins) 1911-1973.
Photo: Kate Hellenbrand

Chapter Three: *The Process*

There are a few die-hard tattooists who still put their sturdy acetate stencils to use and even fewer young artists who, in a desire to pay homage to their forefathers, bring them into service. Supply companies still sell the sheets of plastic, the ground carbon, the carving stylus. (Electric engravers were considered unacceptable by Sailor Jerry, their output lines erratic and choppy.)

Florida tattoo artist Mike Wilson always carries a small Sailor Jerry rose acetate stencil in his wallet. "You never know when someone will want a small rose," he says.

This author, in order to commemorate her mother's recent passing, wanted exactly that small rose; and, as good fortune would have it, esteemed photographer Bill DeMichele was on site to shoot the following sequence:

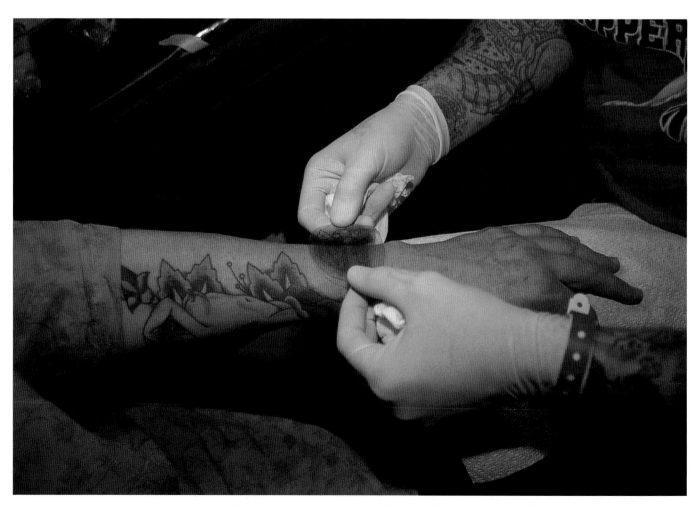

After the client's skin is shaved and moisturized with a thin film of petroleum jelly, the acetate is positioned into place. For these photographs, hectograph (gentian violet) pencil shavings were rubbed into the acetate's grooves rather than the traditional carbon dust.

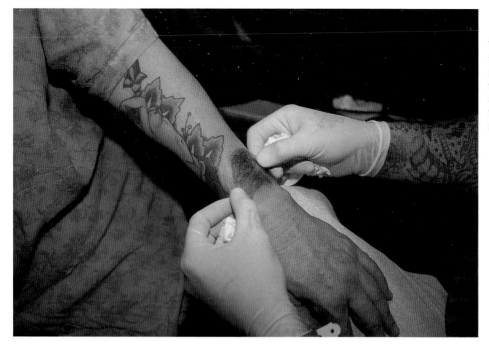

The stencil is then evenly applied to the skin. Too much pressure would smear the design, too little pressure wouldn't leave behind the desired image. Bubbles or any movement under the stencil would also compromise a successful application.

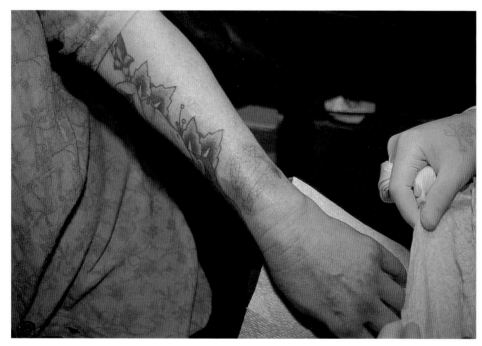

A successful acetate stencil imprint.

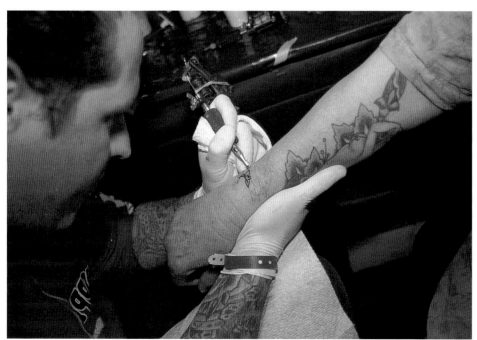

The tattooist then begins to work, usually from the right or left hand corner and up into the design. A well-functioning machine is vital at this point. Care must be taken not to disturb the remainder of the stencil outline as the work is being done.

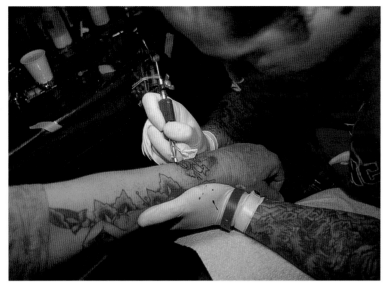

Finally, the tattoo outline is finished at the top of the design.

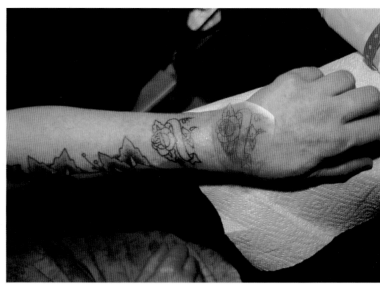

An absolutely accurate outline of the desired design.

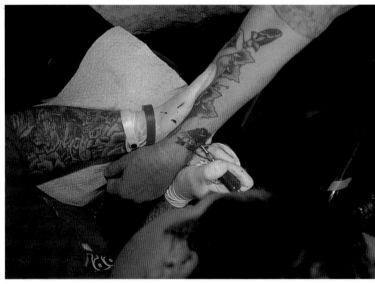

Now for the color, usually progressing up through the color wheel in order of darkest to lightest. In the acetate's heyday, only three or four colors were available: black, red, green, and sometimes yellow.

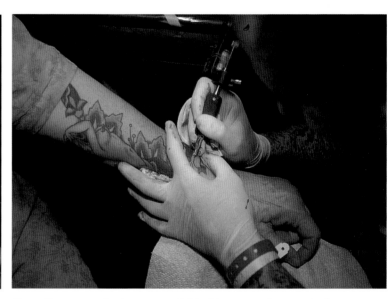

Currently, scores of colors are available. Here a small amount of blue is added for background depth.

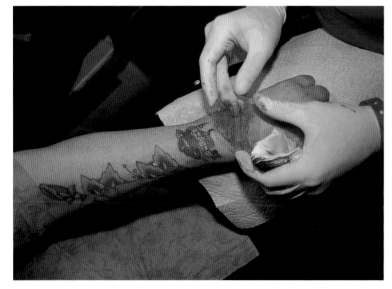

There you have it, a beautiful little Sailor Jerry rose. Bright, solid, and built to last a lifetime.

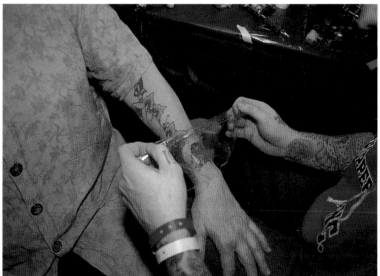

The tattoo is protected for the first stage of healing. An application of ointment, a see-through covering of plastic will suffice until a lymph (scab) covering is generated by the body's own defense mechanism. The development of a new dermal layer of skin over the fields of pigment will take 7 to 10 days.

Chapter Four: *The Stencils*

The designs in this book are computer-scanned from actual Sailor Jerry Collins acetate and celluloid tattoo stencils. All imperfections and markings are seen here. Each stencil is seen exact size and in the same condition as the day Jerry died in 1973. Some stencils were moderately to heavily used and the blurry lines are from the residual carbon dust still in the grooves. These stencils have not been cleaned or altered in any way.

Each stencil is signed by Jerry, either with a commingled NKC, SJ, his famous stamp, or signed name. NKC stands for Sailor Jerry's given name: Norman Keith Collins. He signed his stencils with this symbol until the late 1960s. SJ was adopted by Sailor Jerry in the late 1960s. Sometimes he coupled the initials so they resembled a dollar sign. Sailor Jerry also used a stamp or would sign his acetates with Jerry or Sailor Jerry. The stencils were always signed on the reverse side of the design so the tattoo would not be inadvertently signed. Other marks on the stencils would relate to Jerry's filing system.

In the great tradition of tattoo design presentation in shops around the world since the beginning of the business, these stencil images are not necessarily categorized or grouped together in any logical fashion. They are, instead, put together in "pork sheet" style, randomly, without reason. In this way, each design is a happy discovery. Enjoy.

Due to Sailor Jerry's still increasing fame, inquiries should be made as to the current price and availability. Please address the author at 274 9th Street #3, Brooklyn, NY 11215. Phone numbers: 718-369-4893 or 917-446-9909. Email: dameoftheworld@aol.com

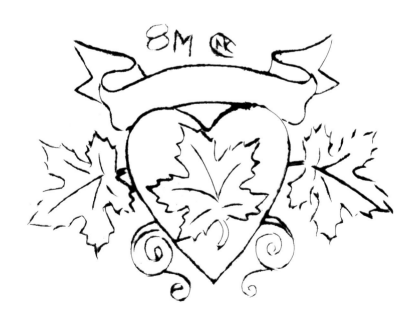

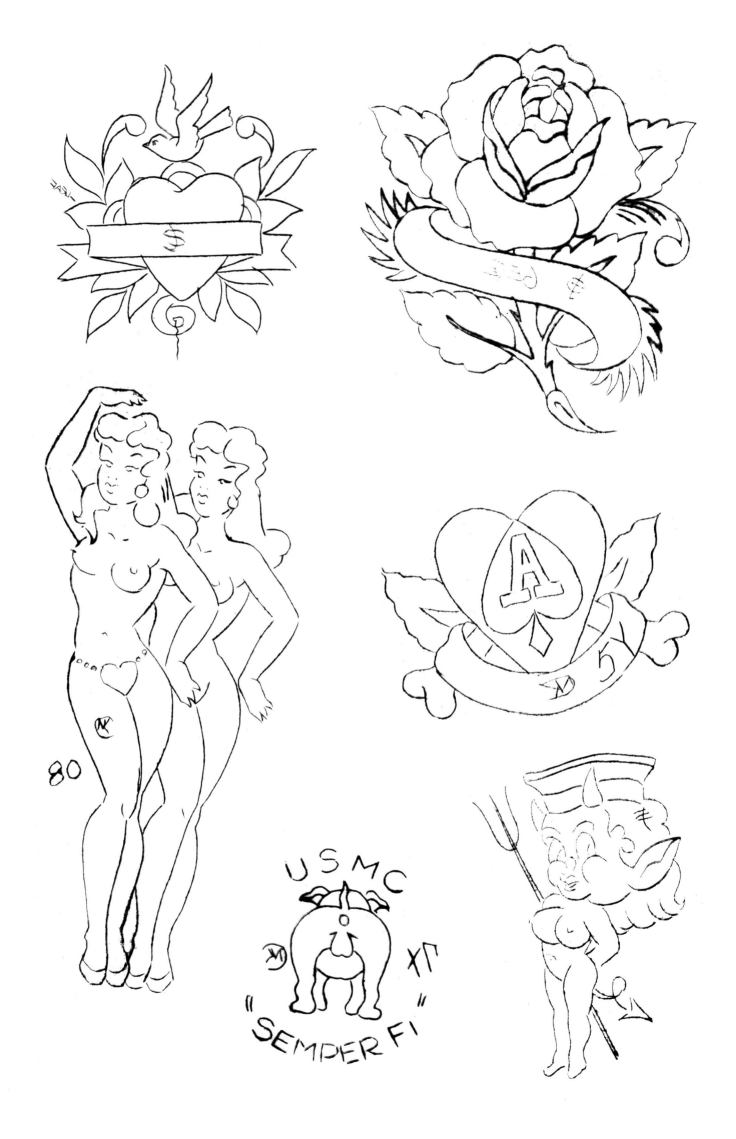

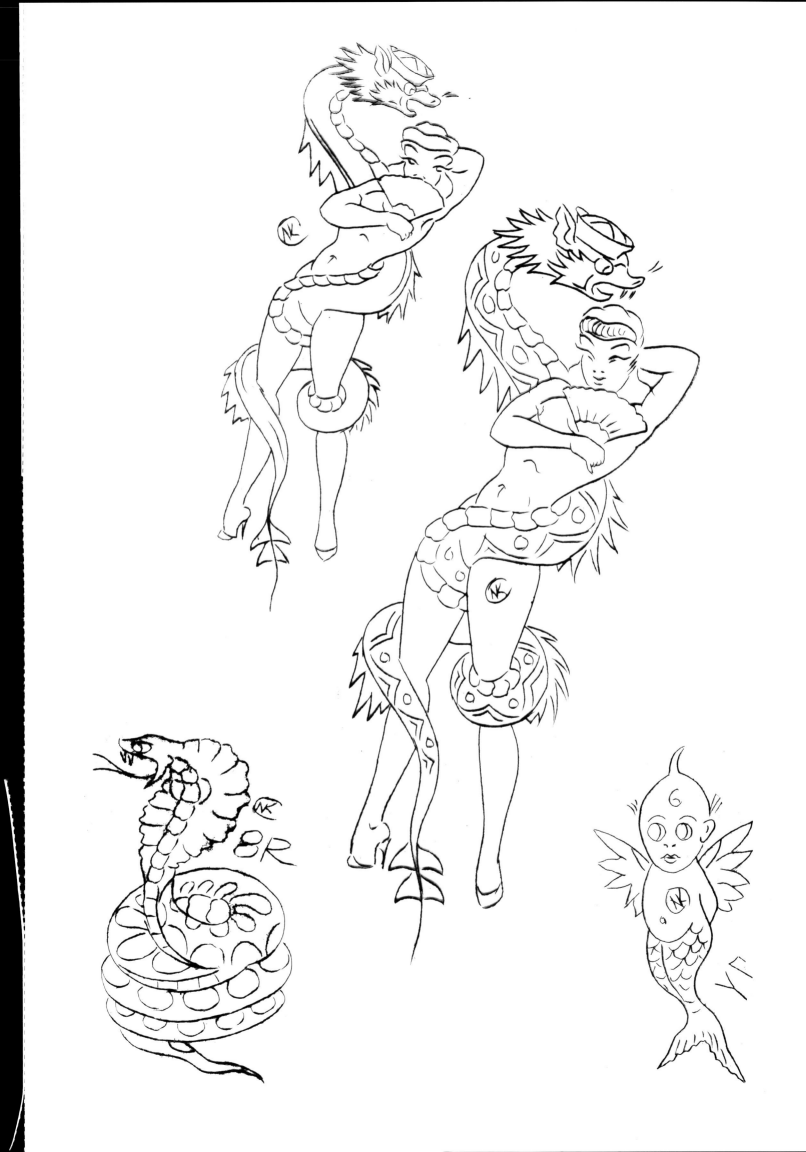

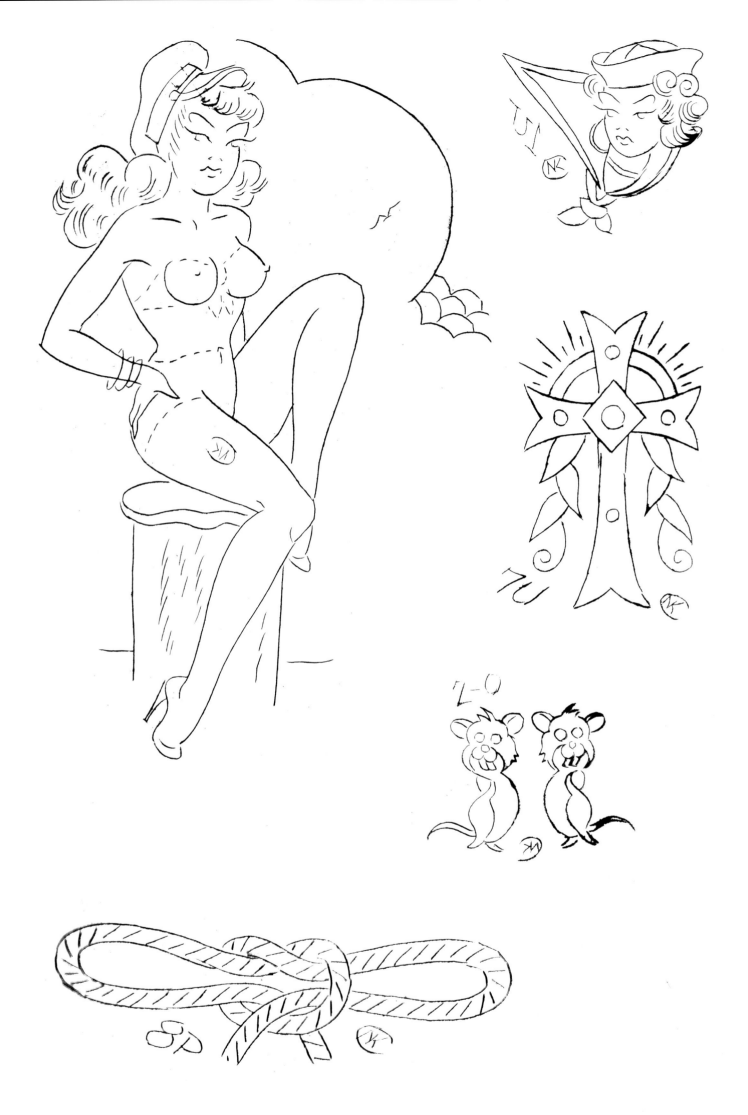

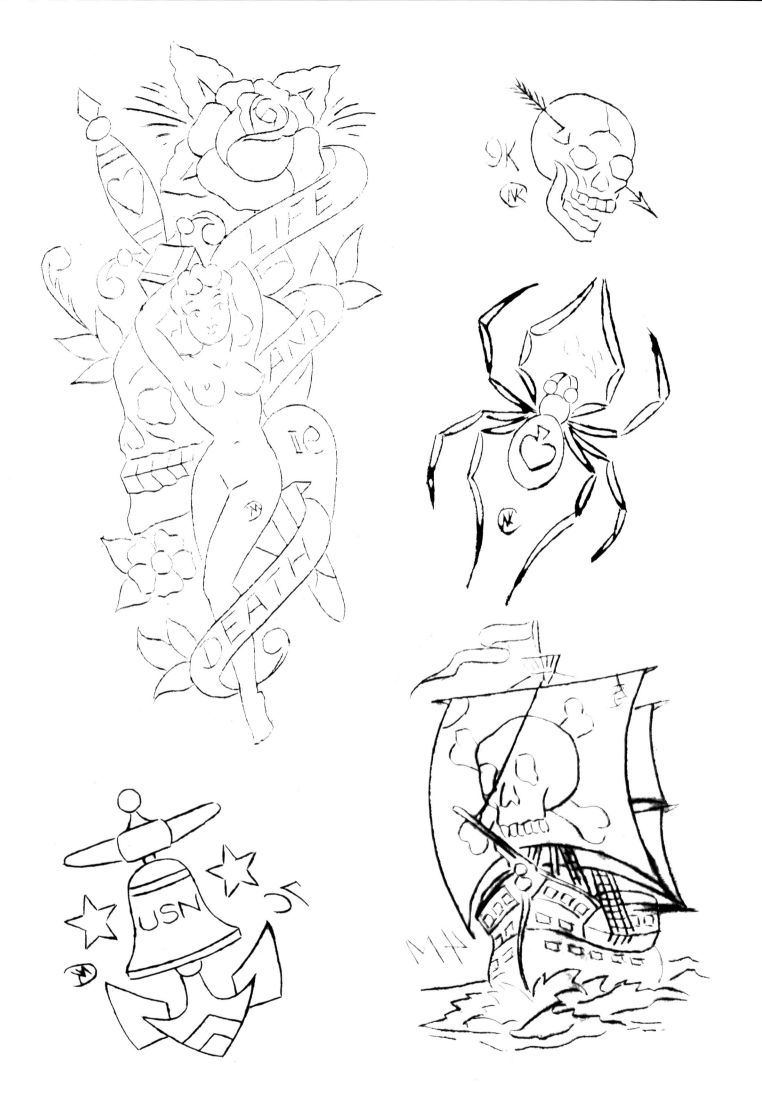

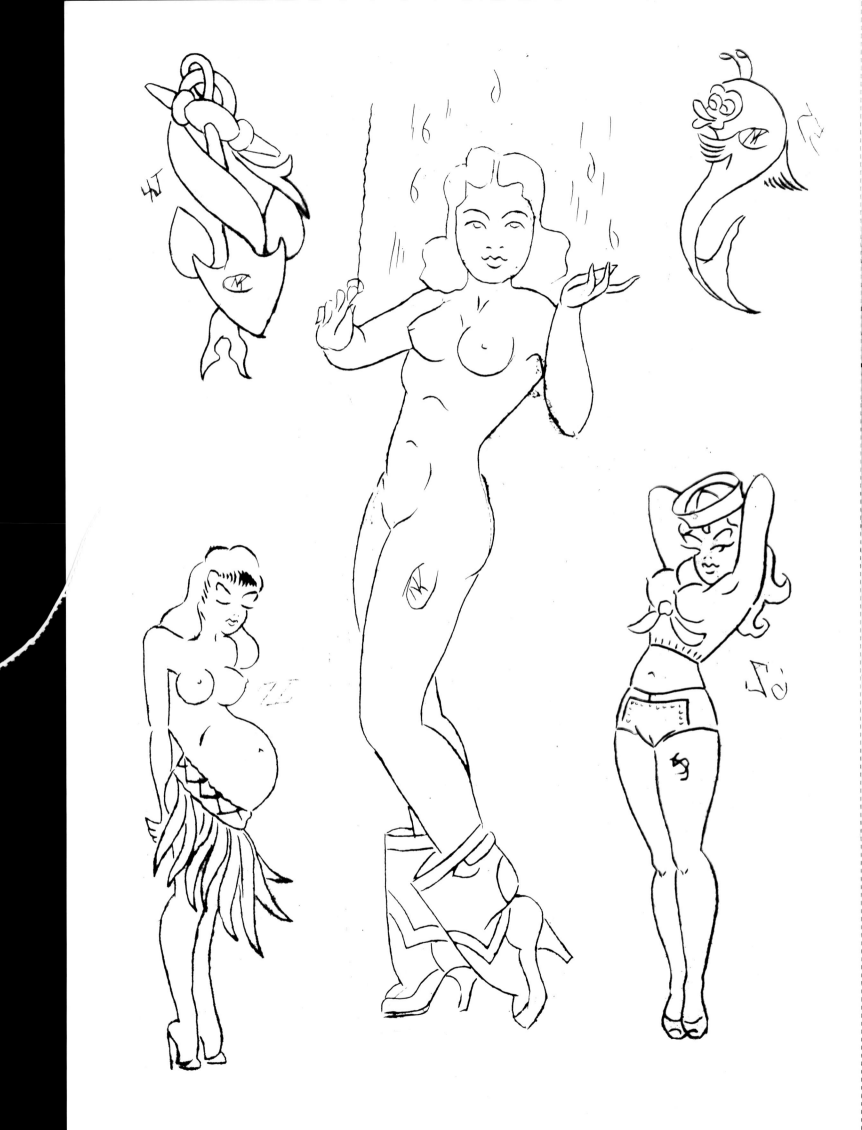

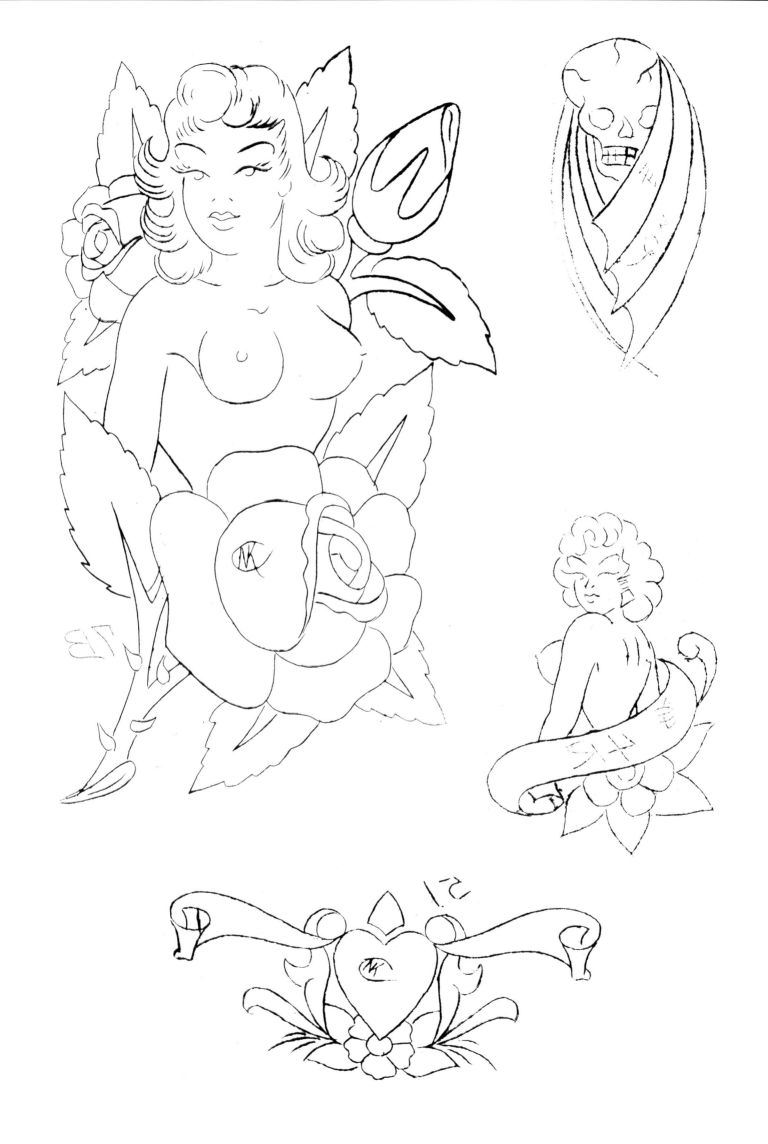

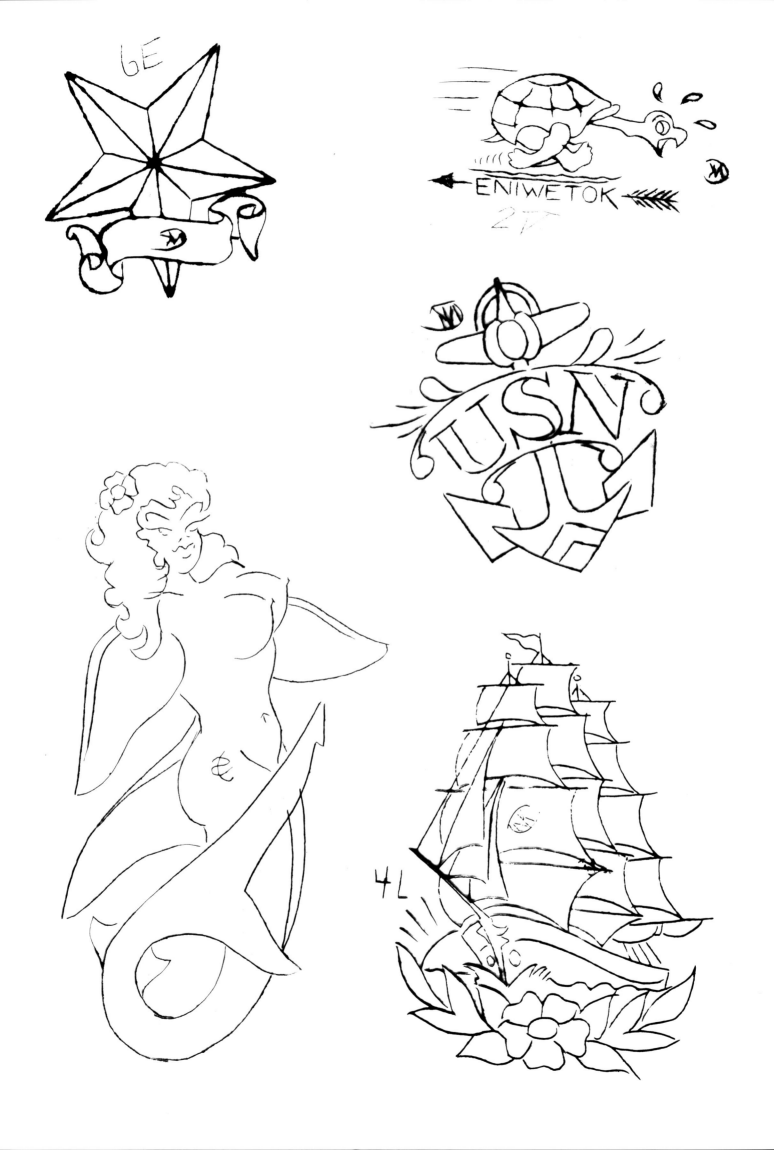

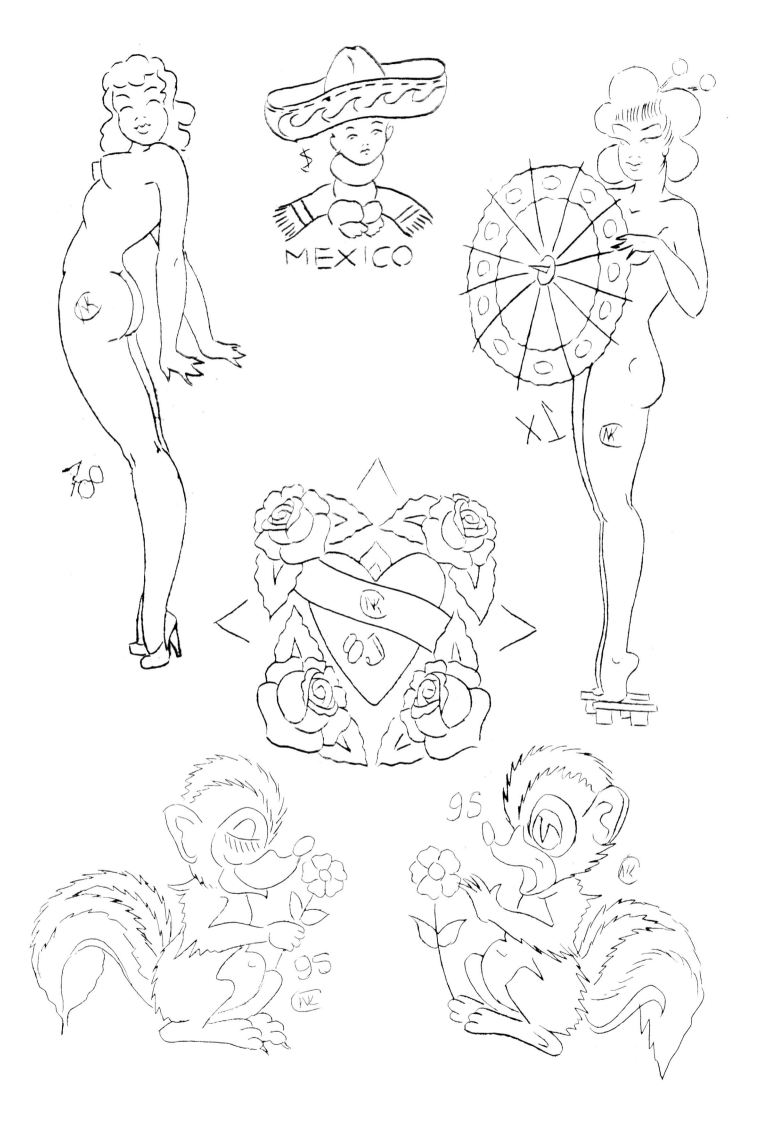

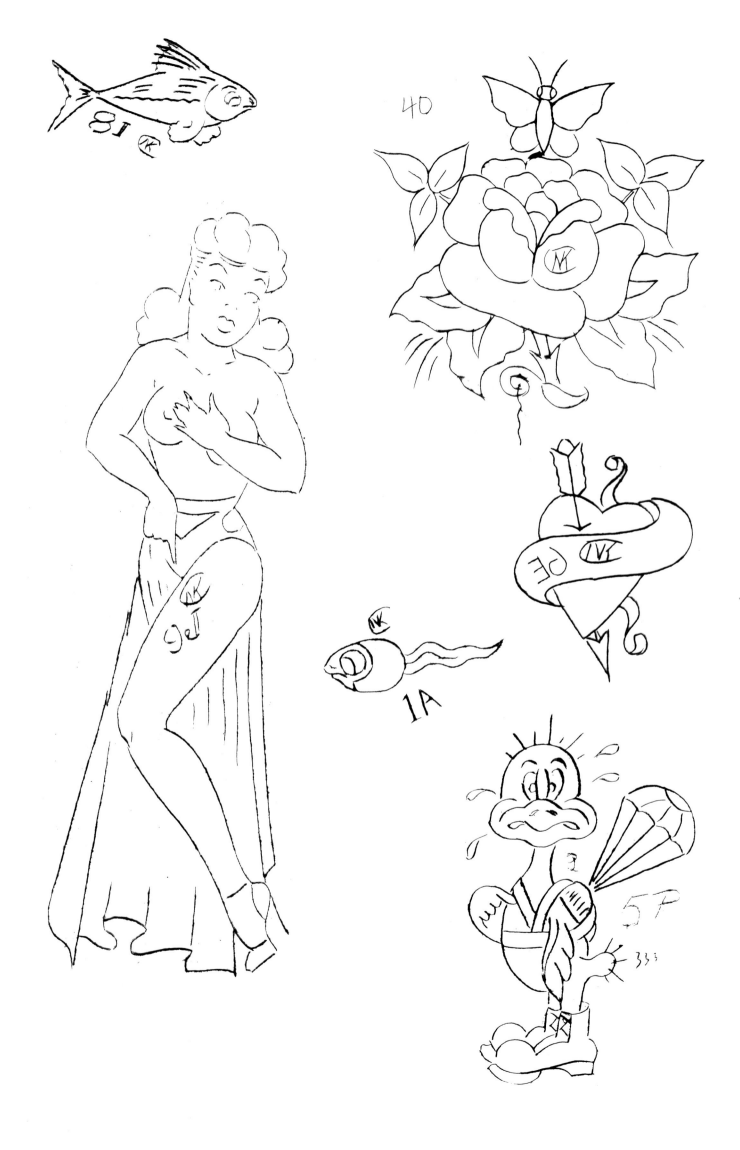

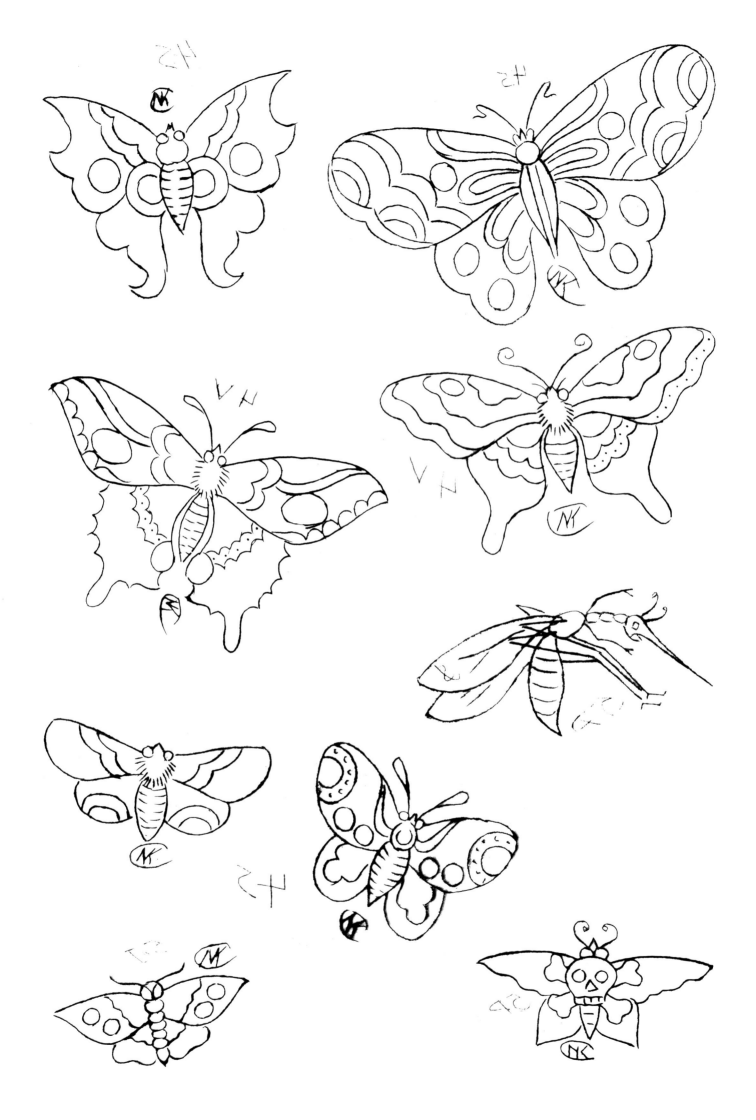

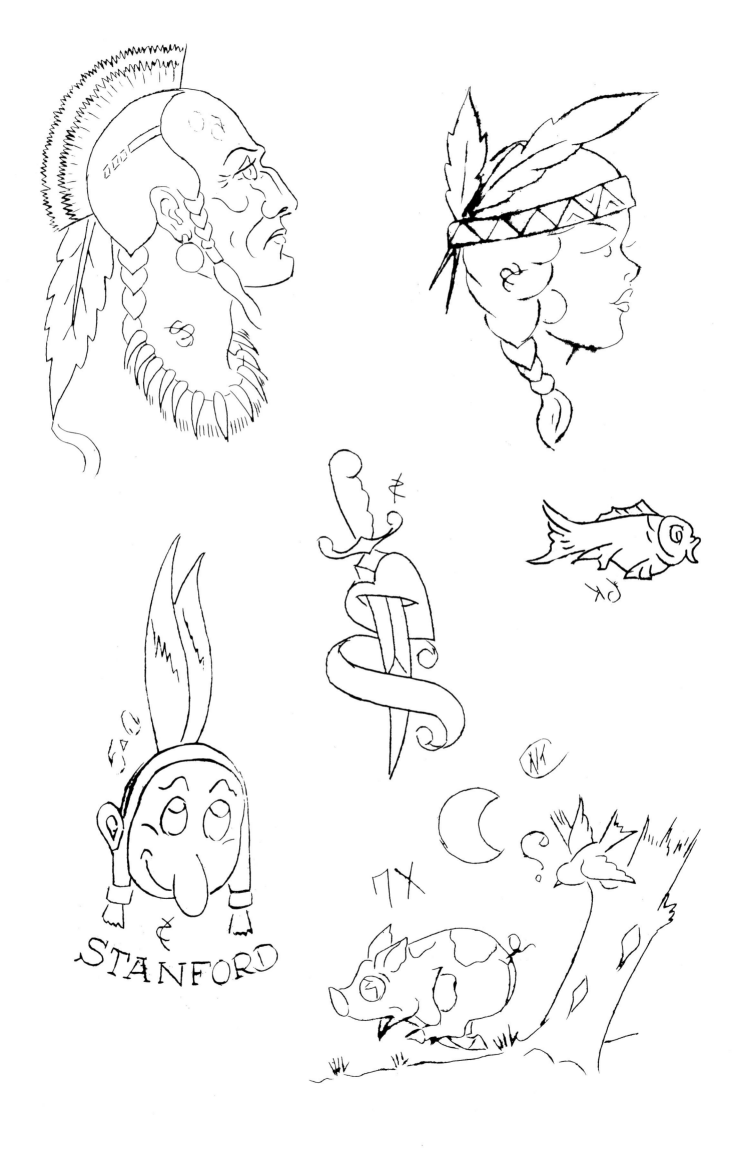

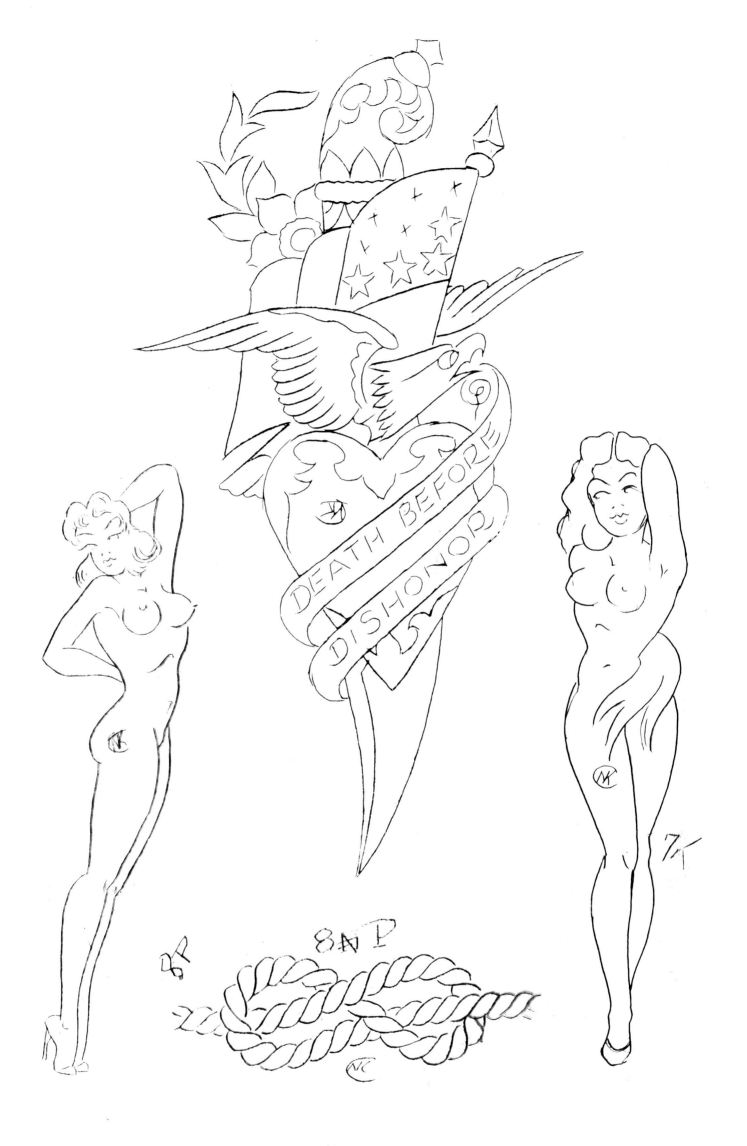

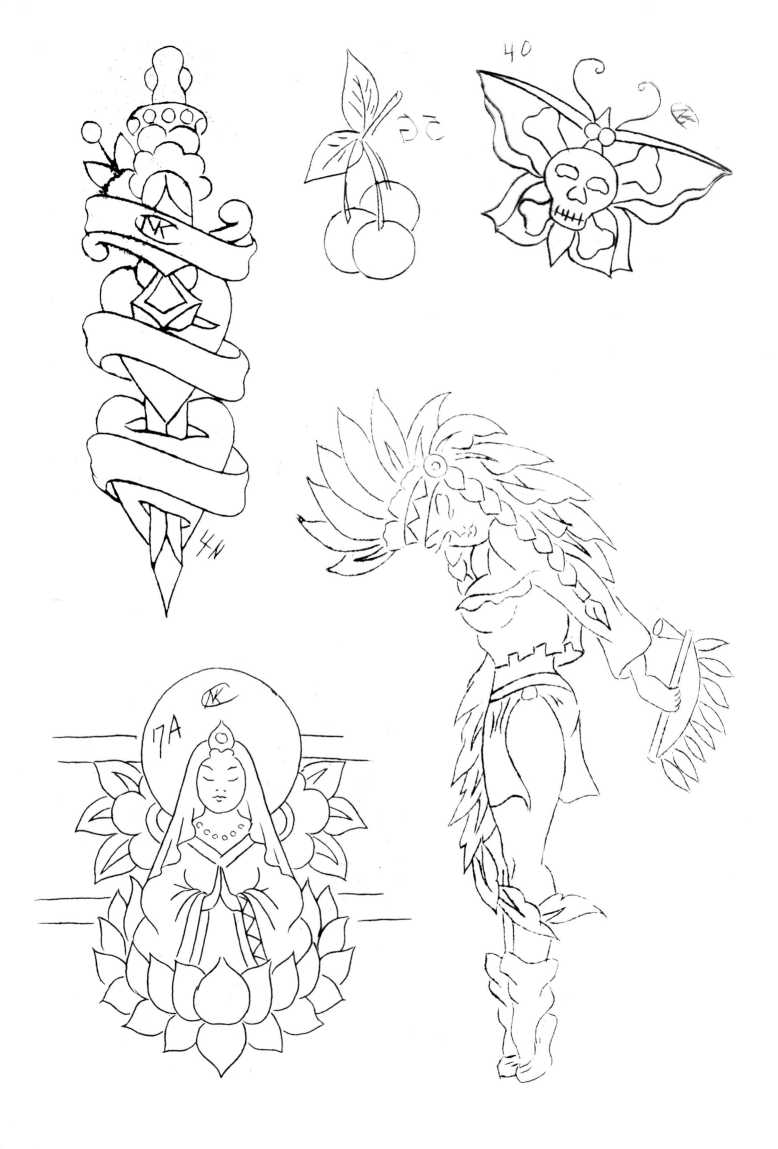

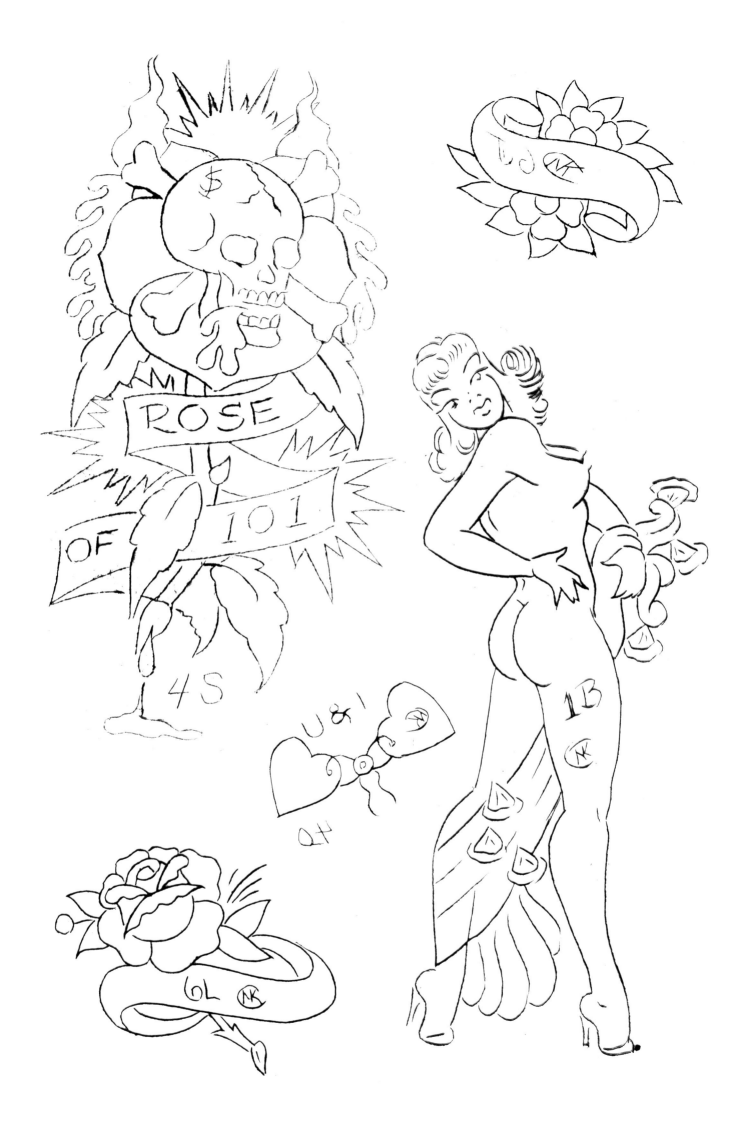

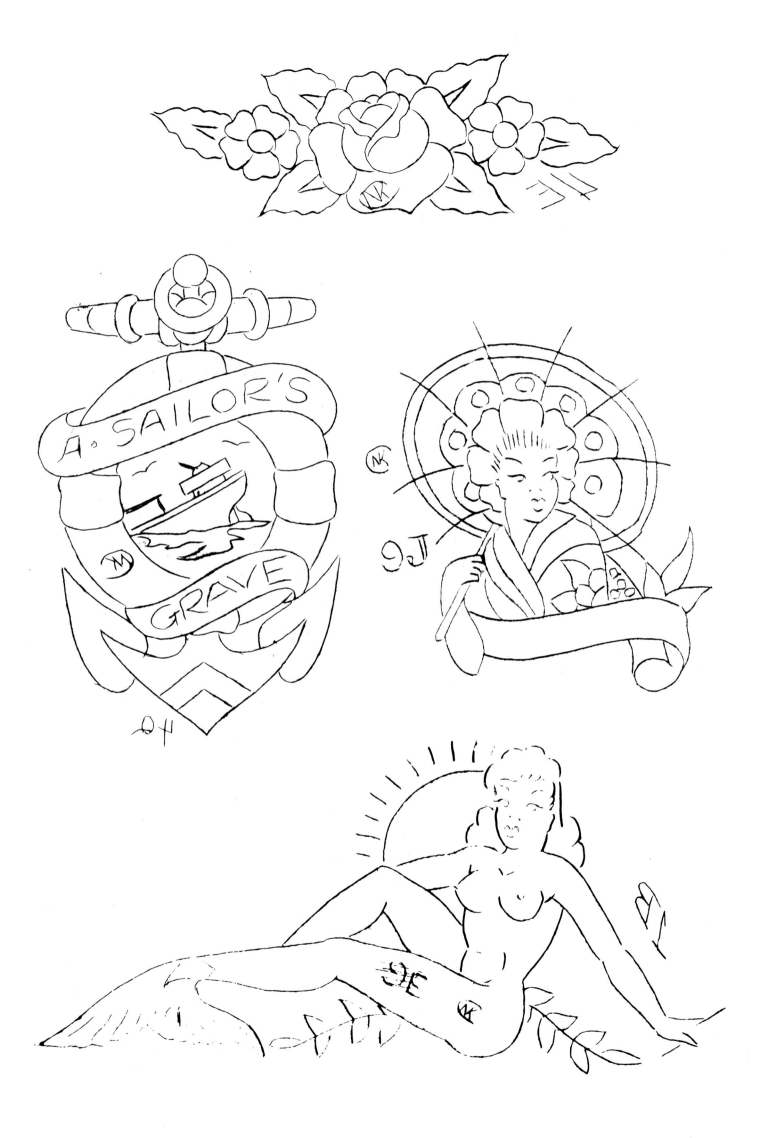

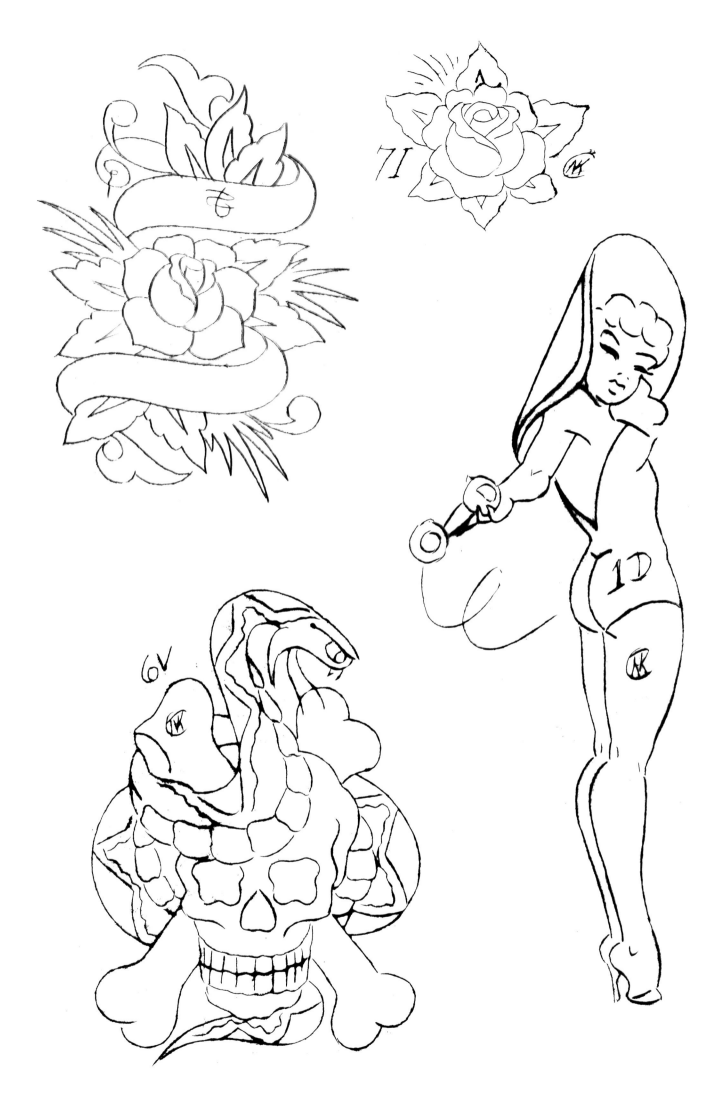

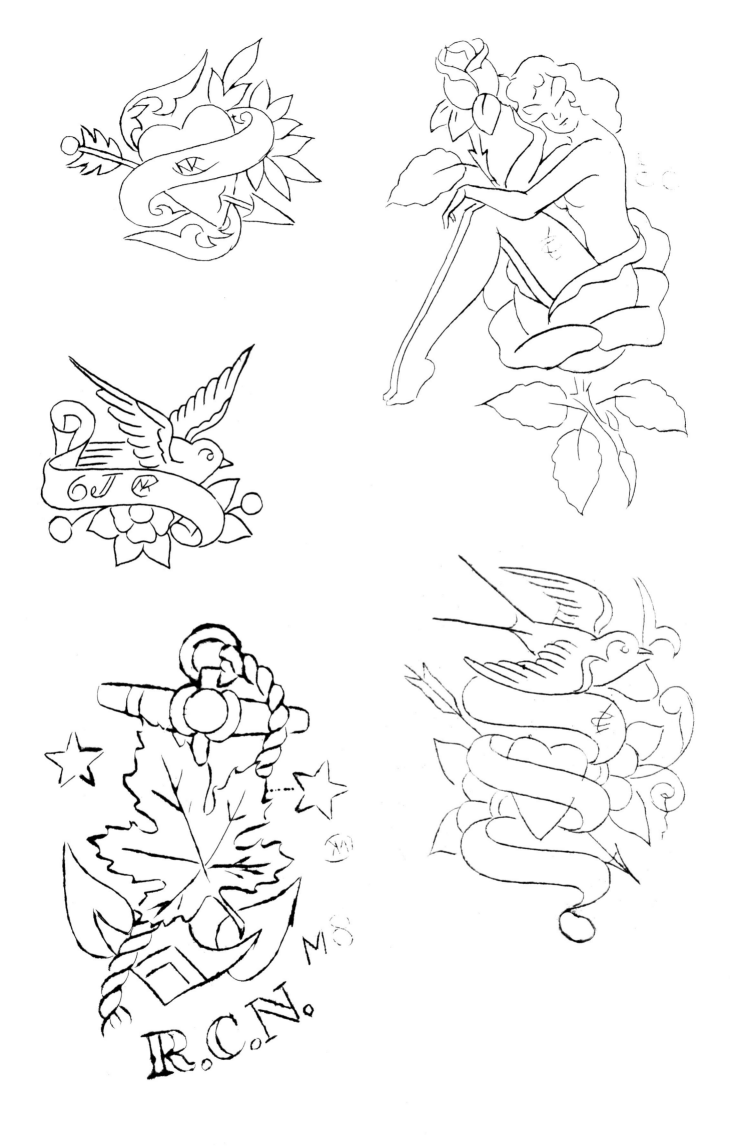

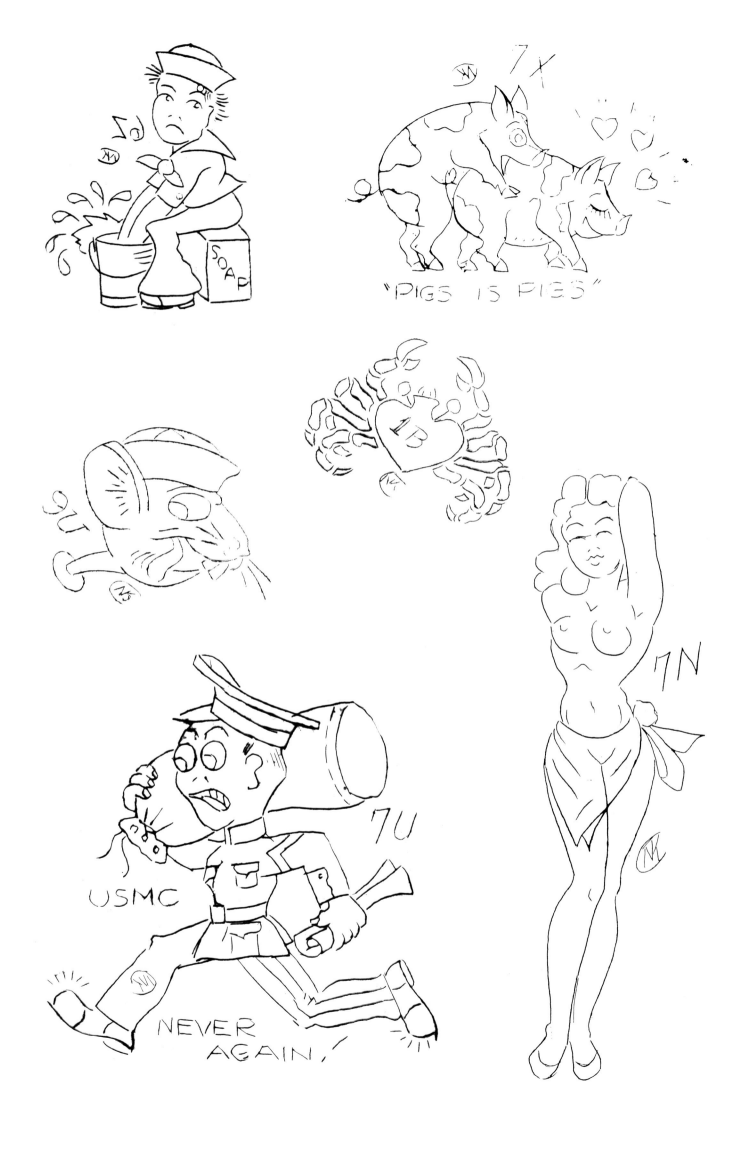

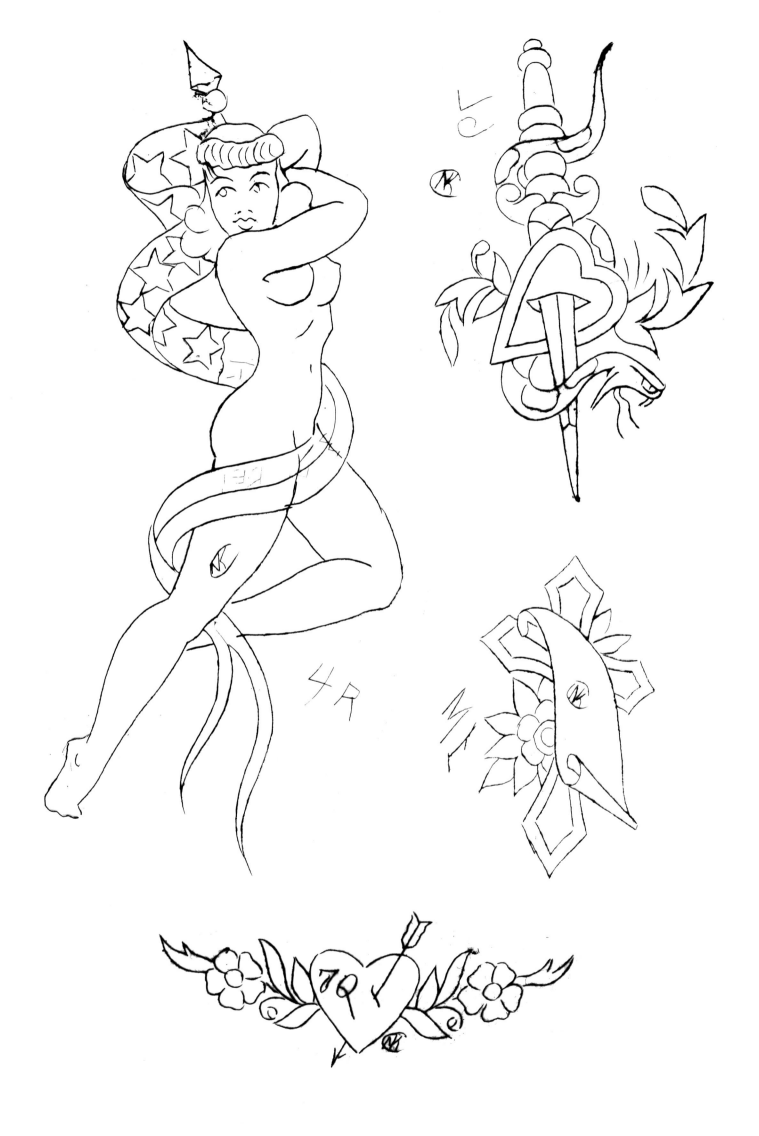

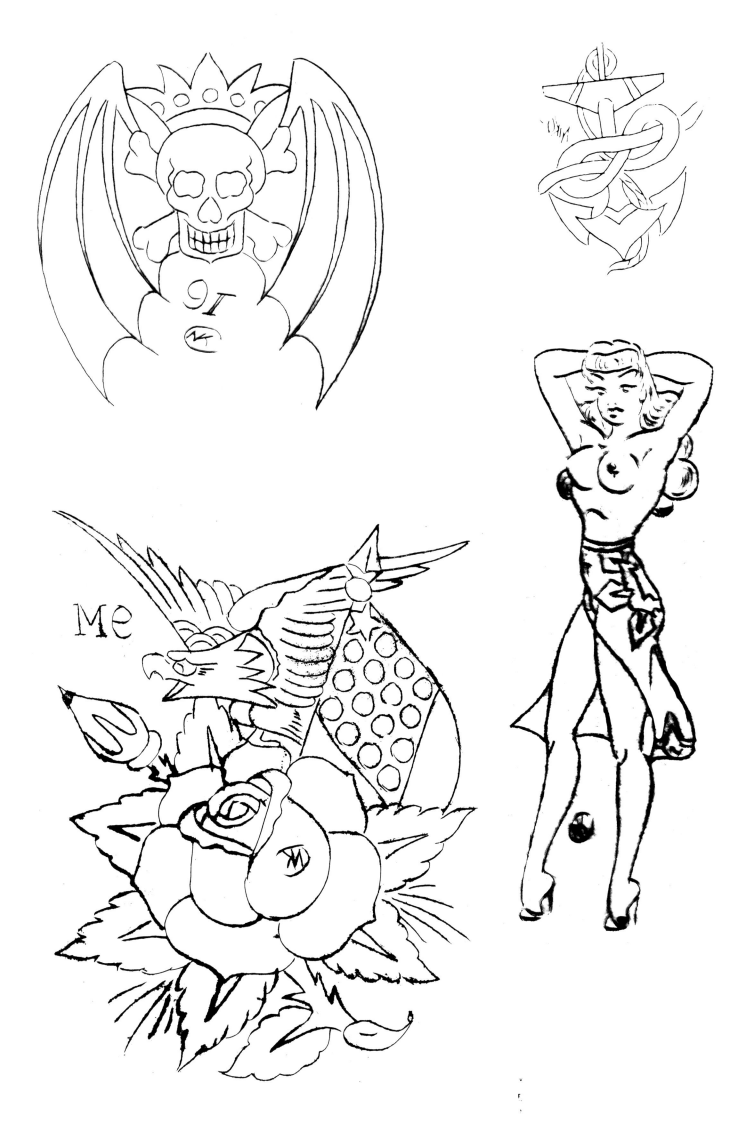

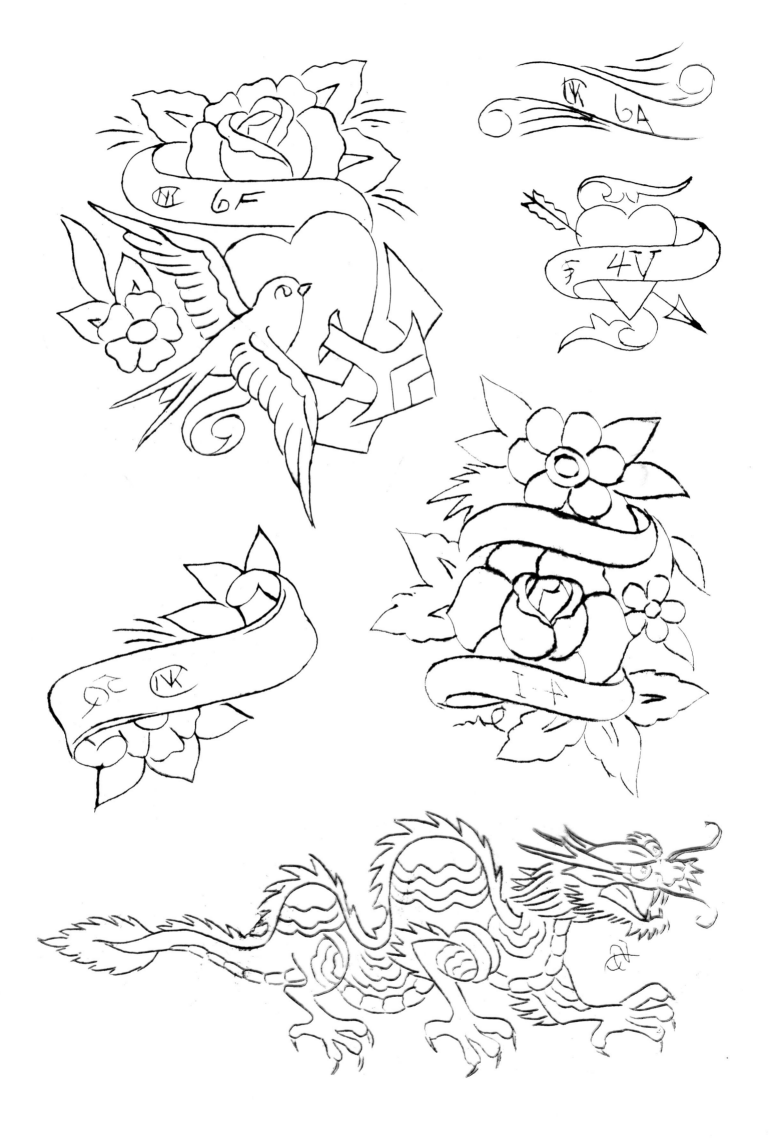

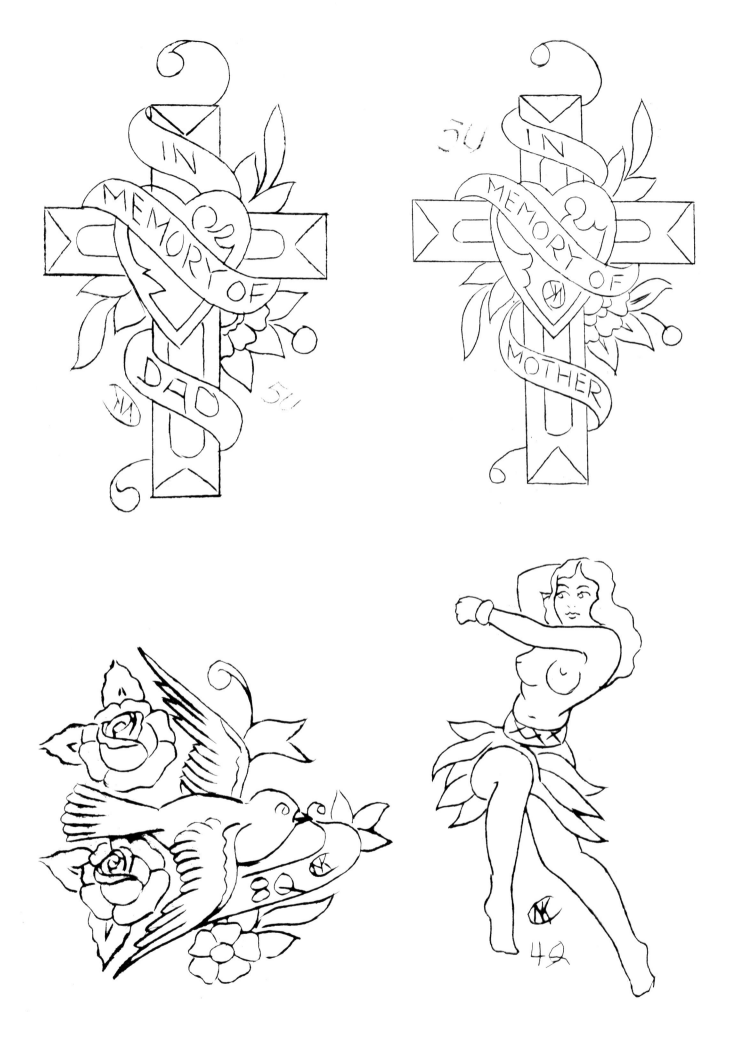

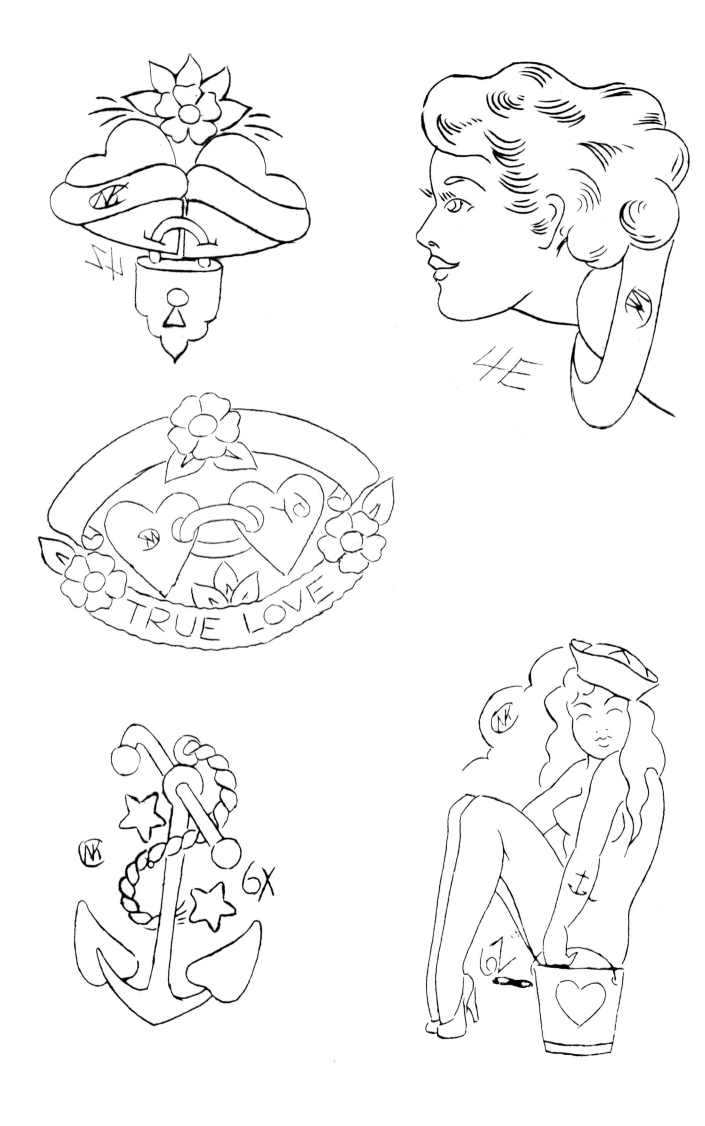

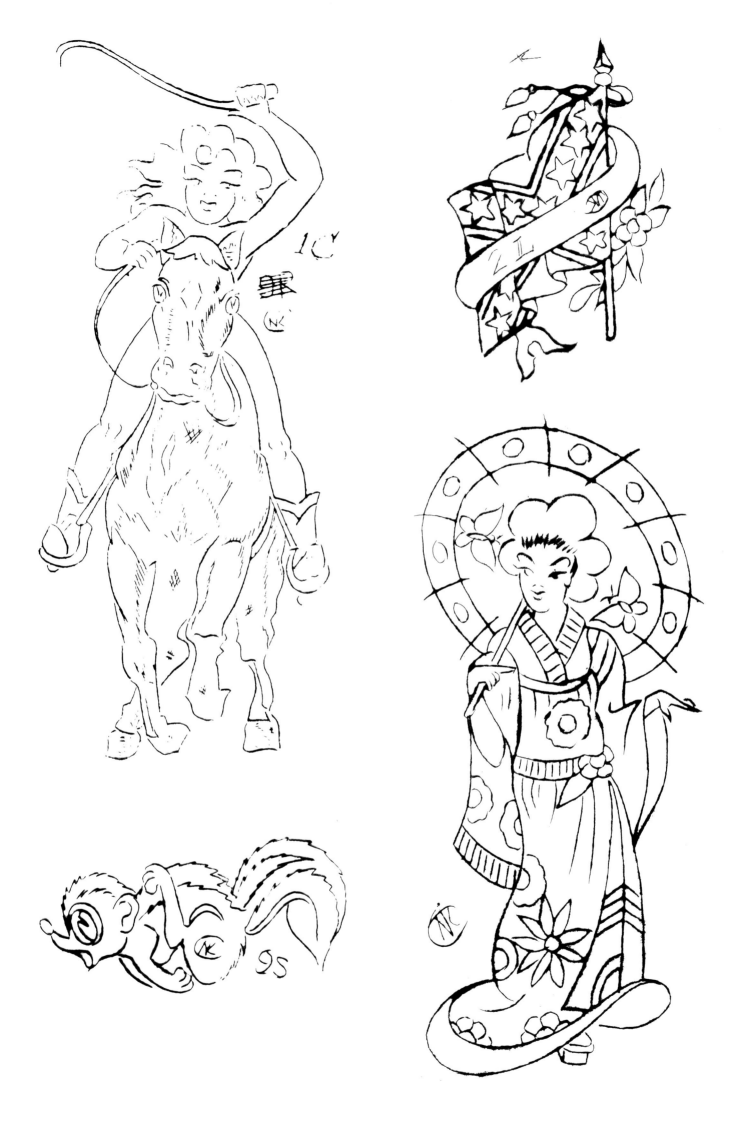

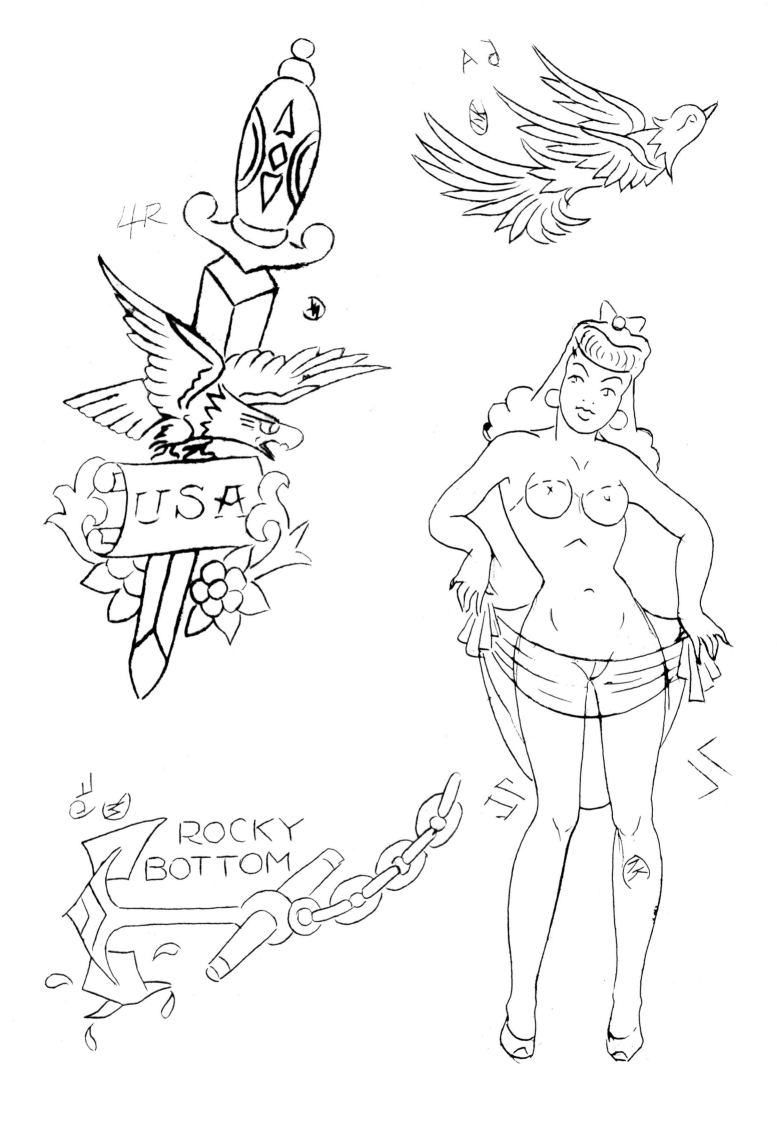

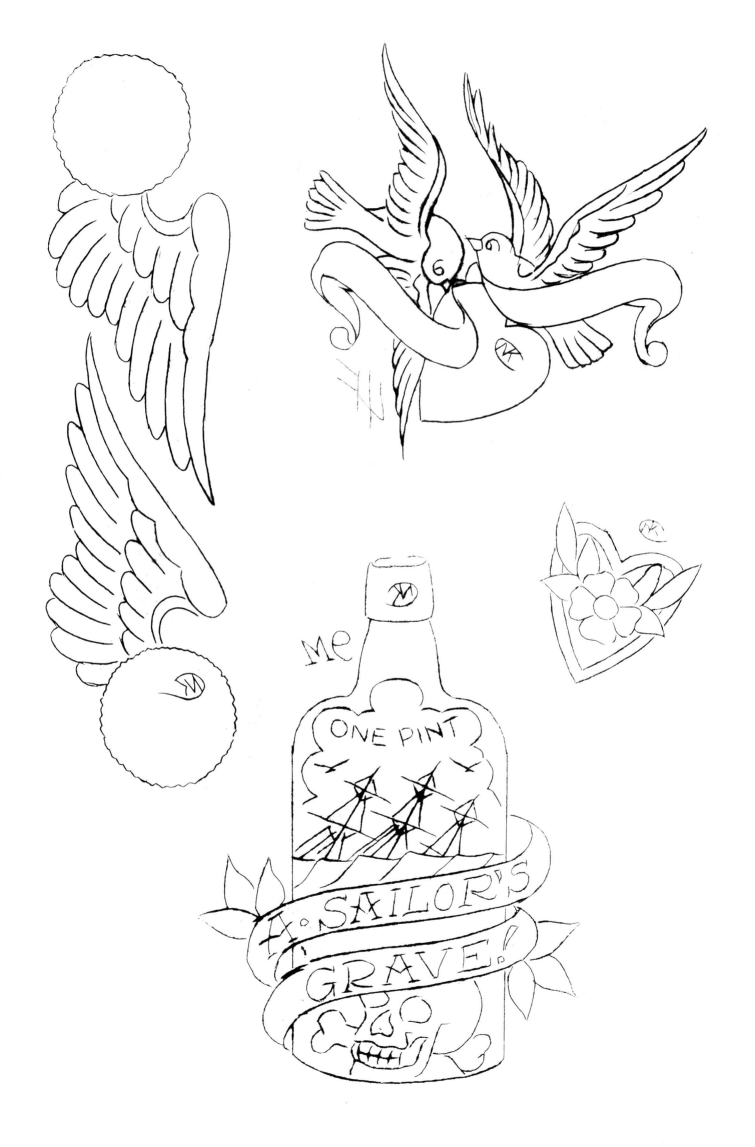

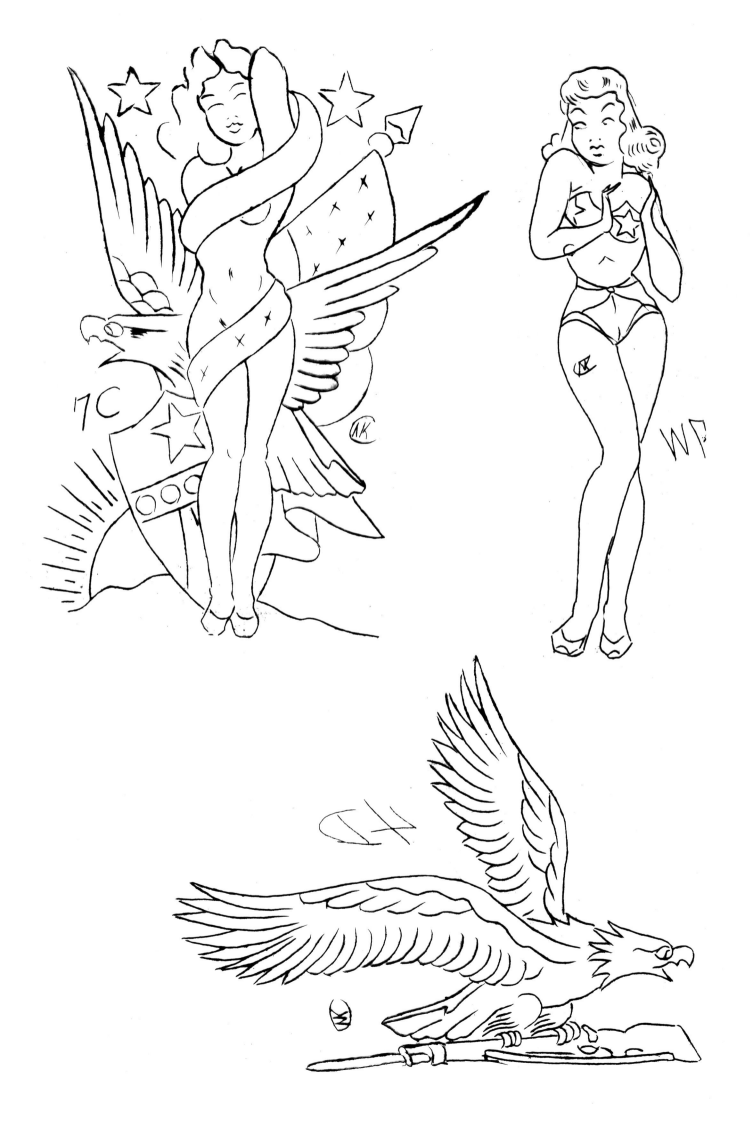

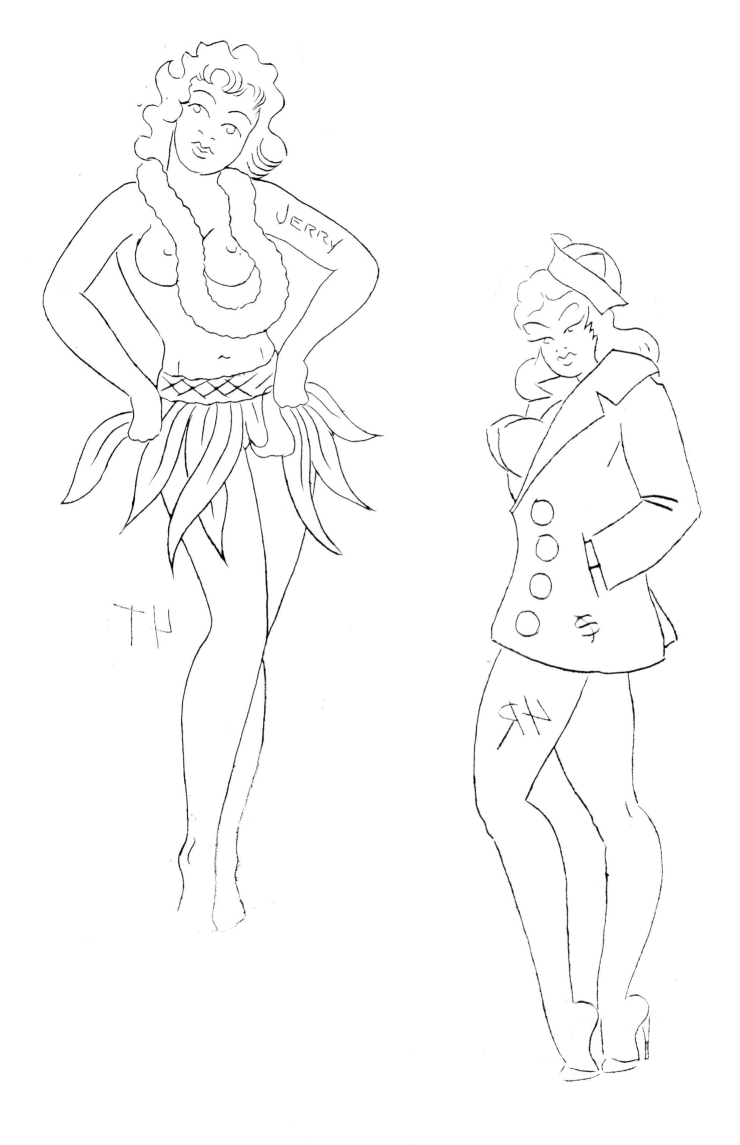

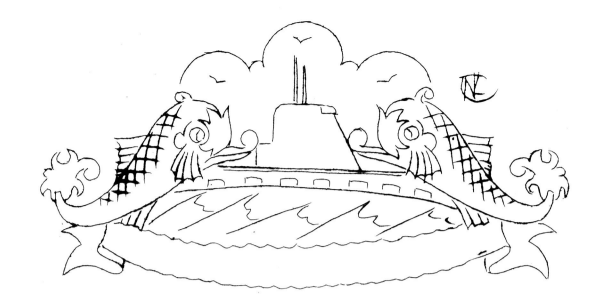

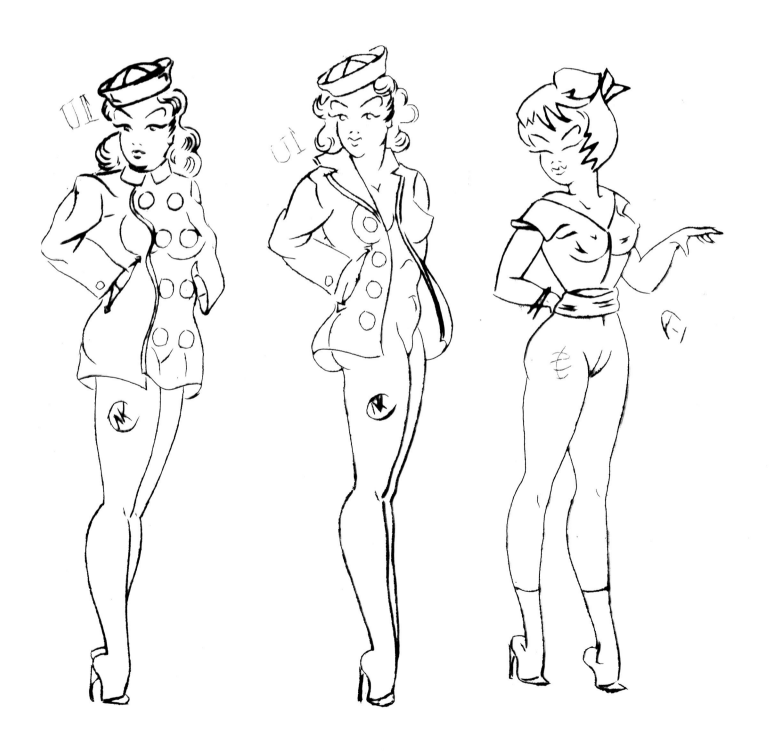

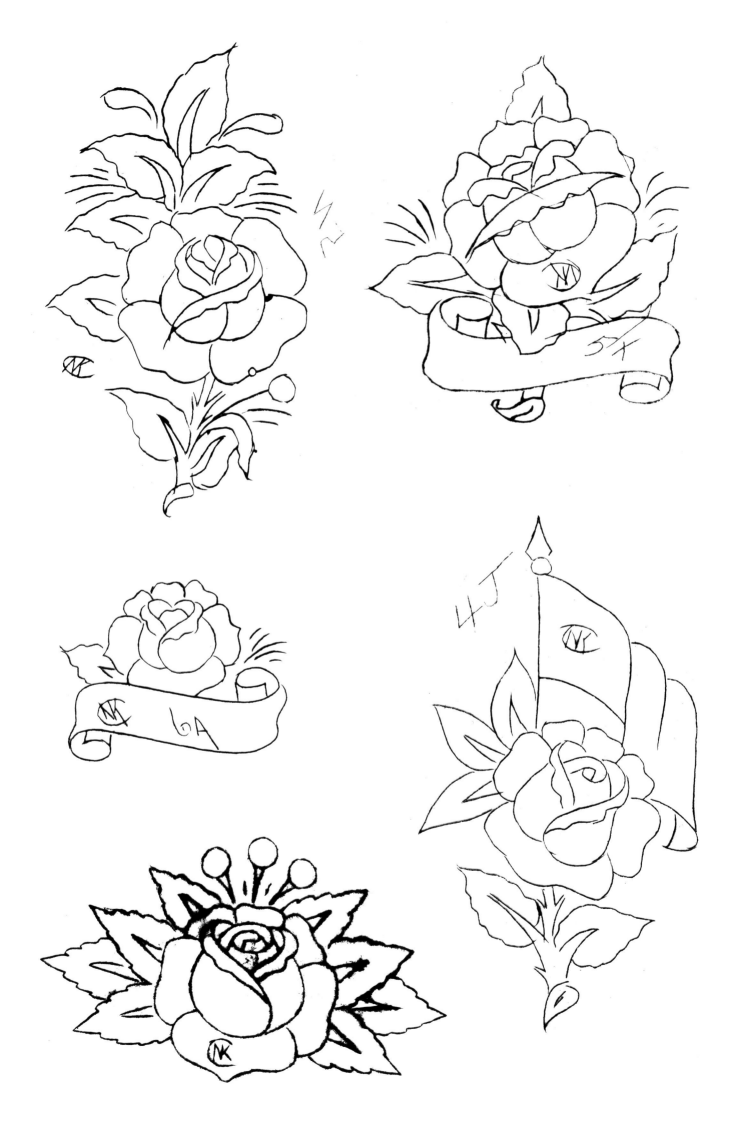

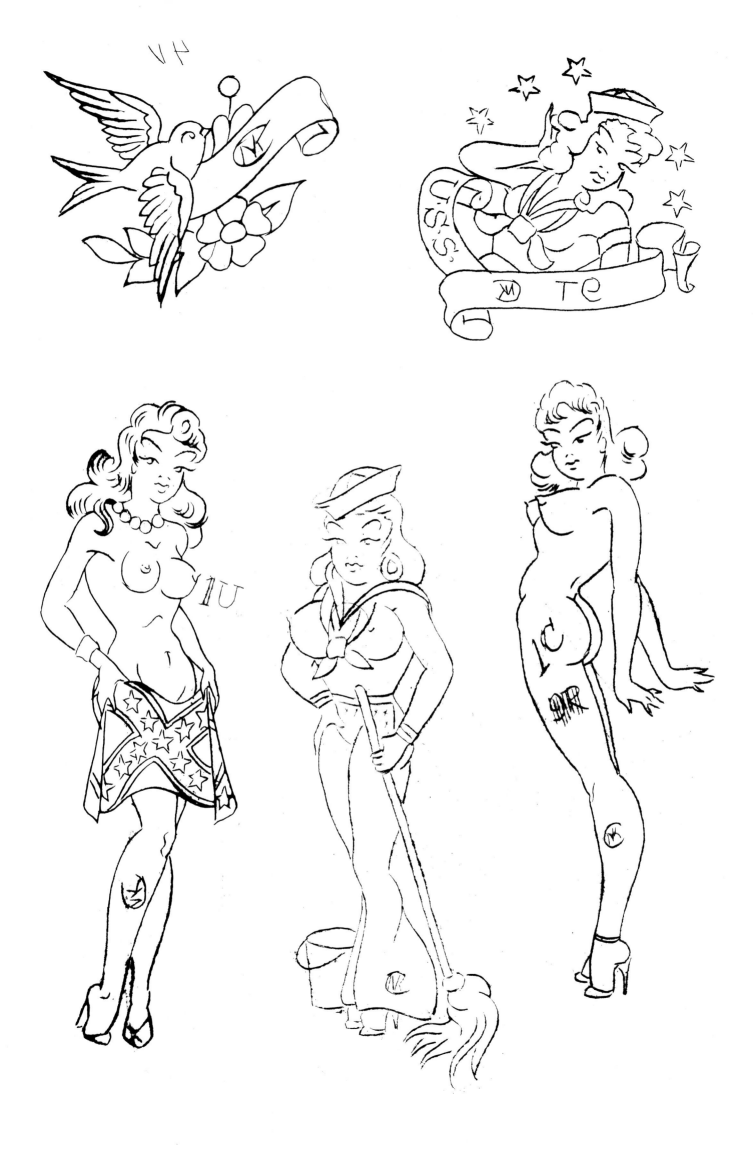

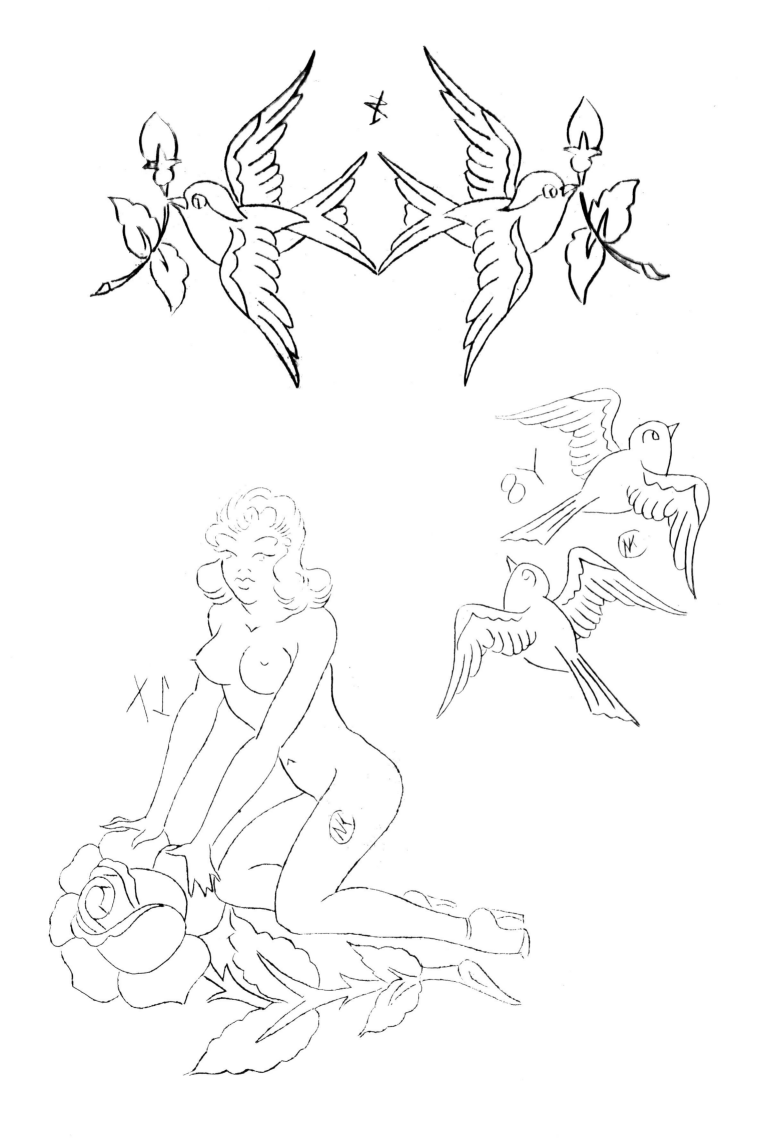

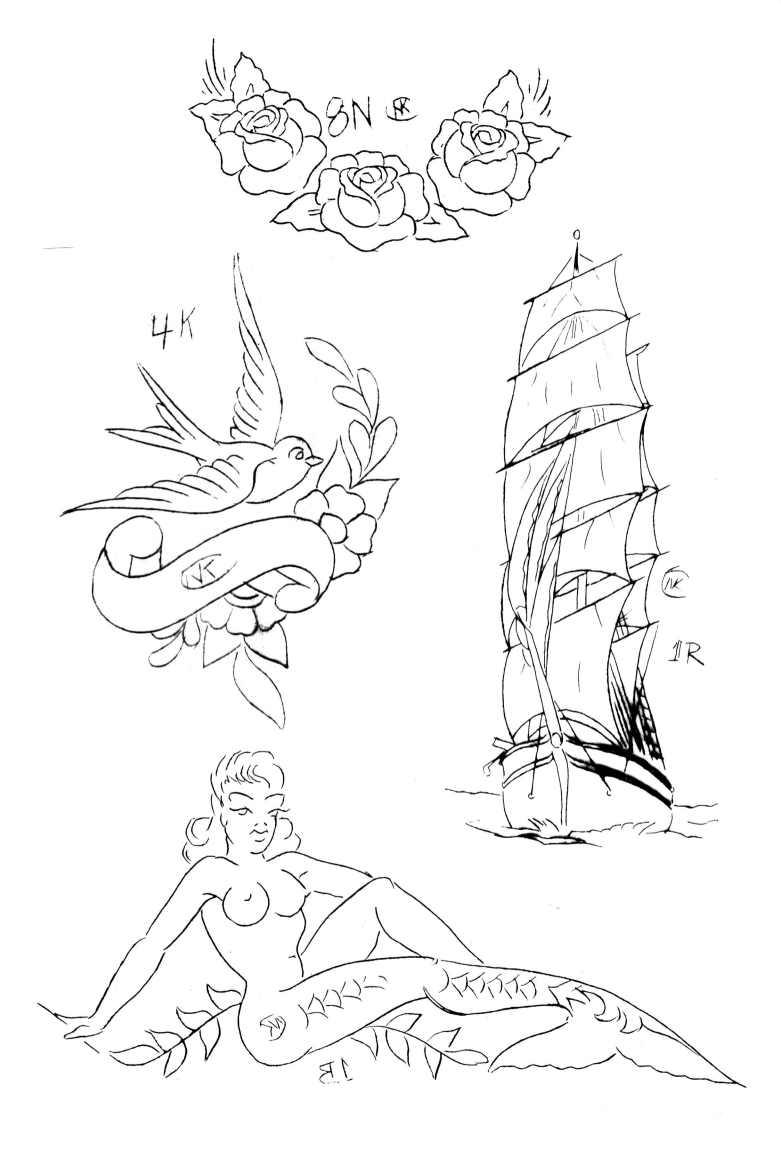

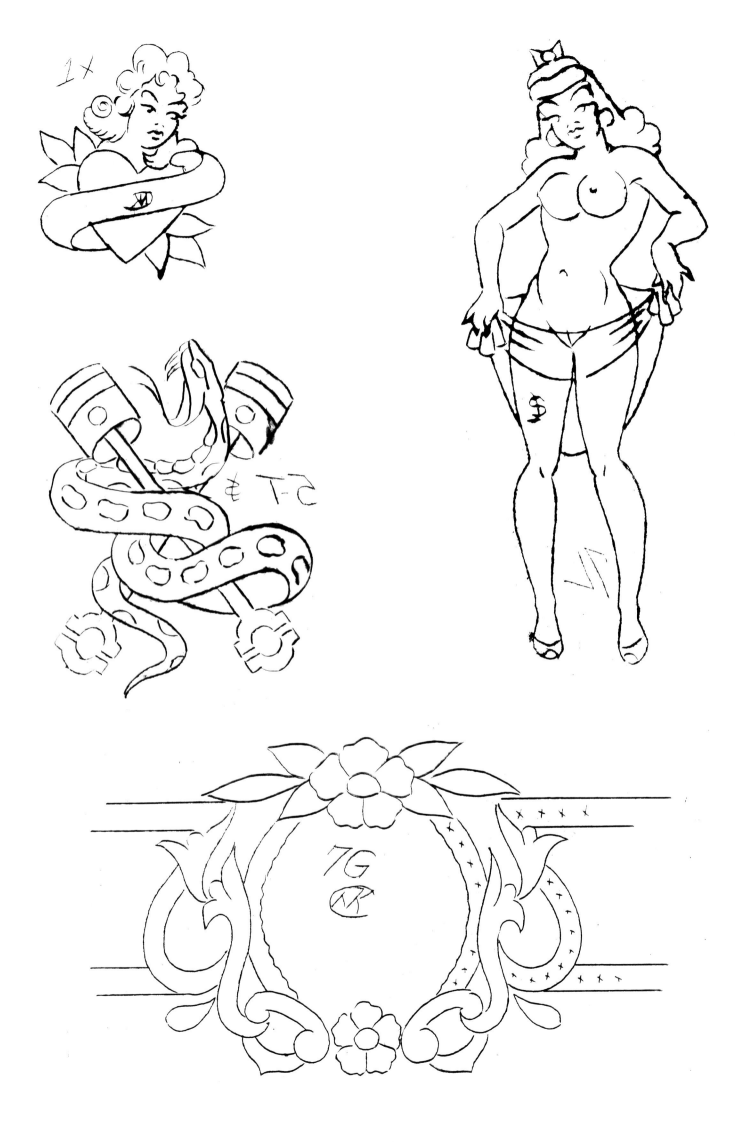

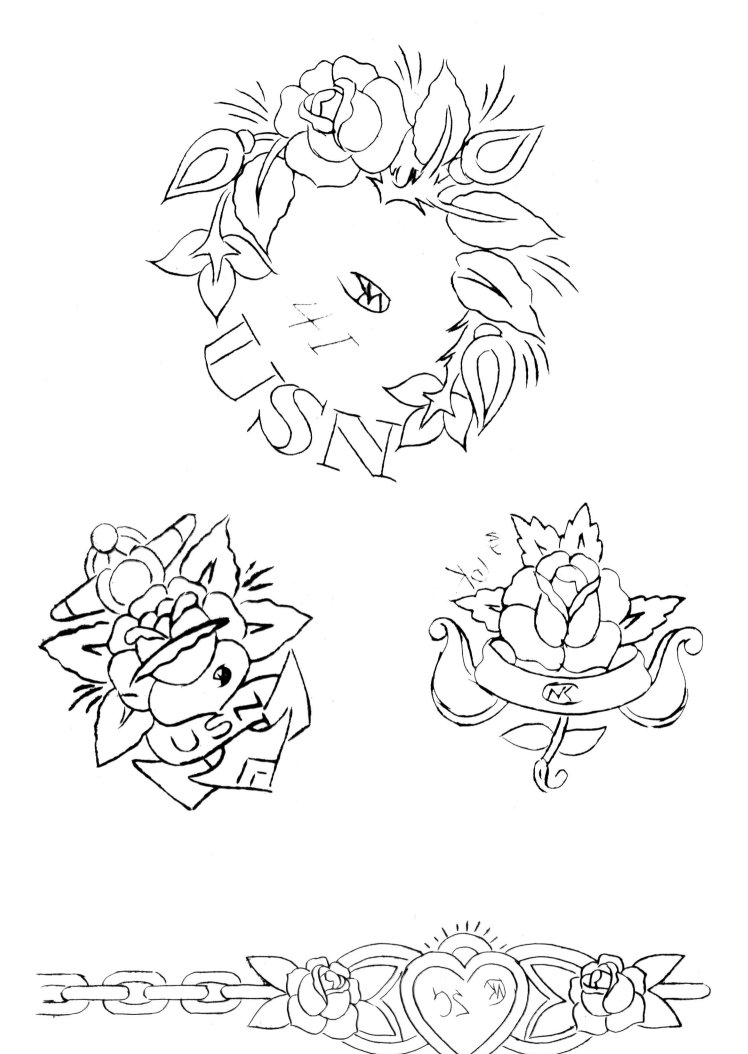

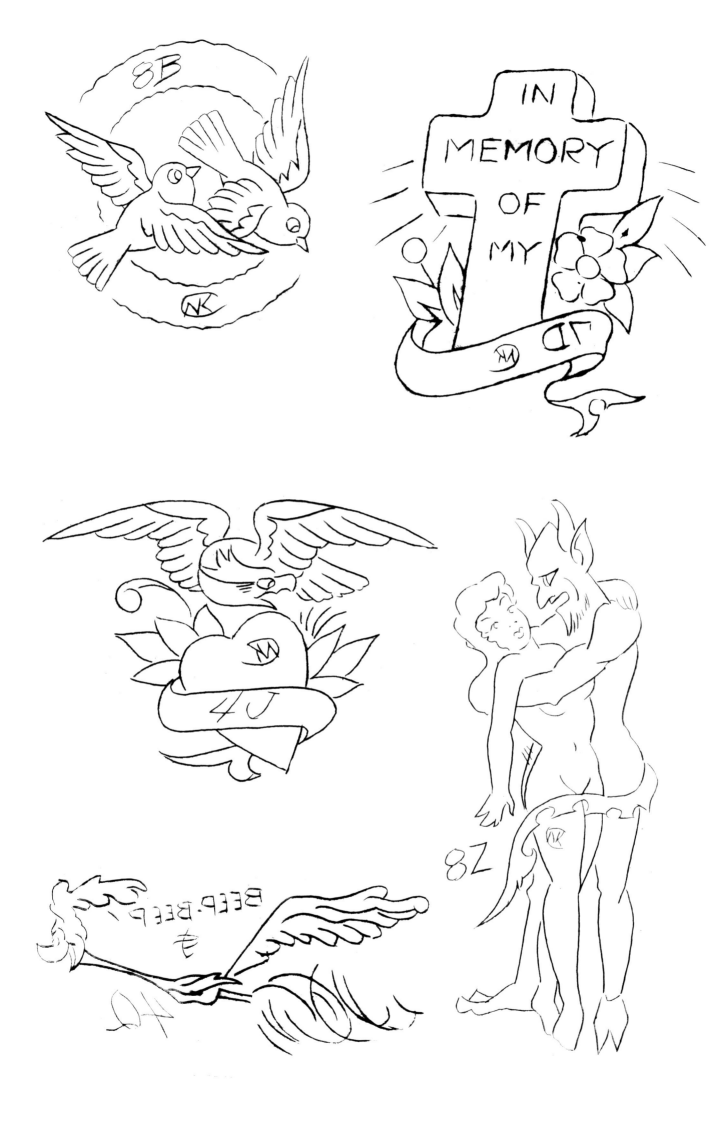

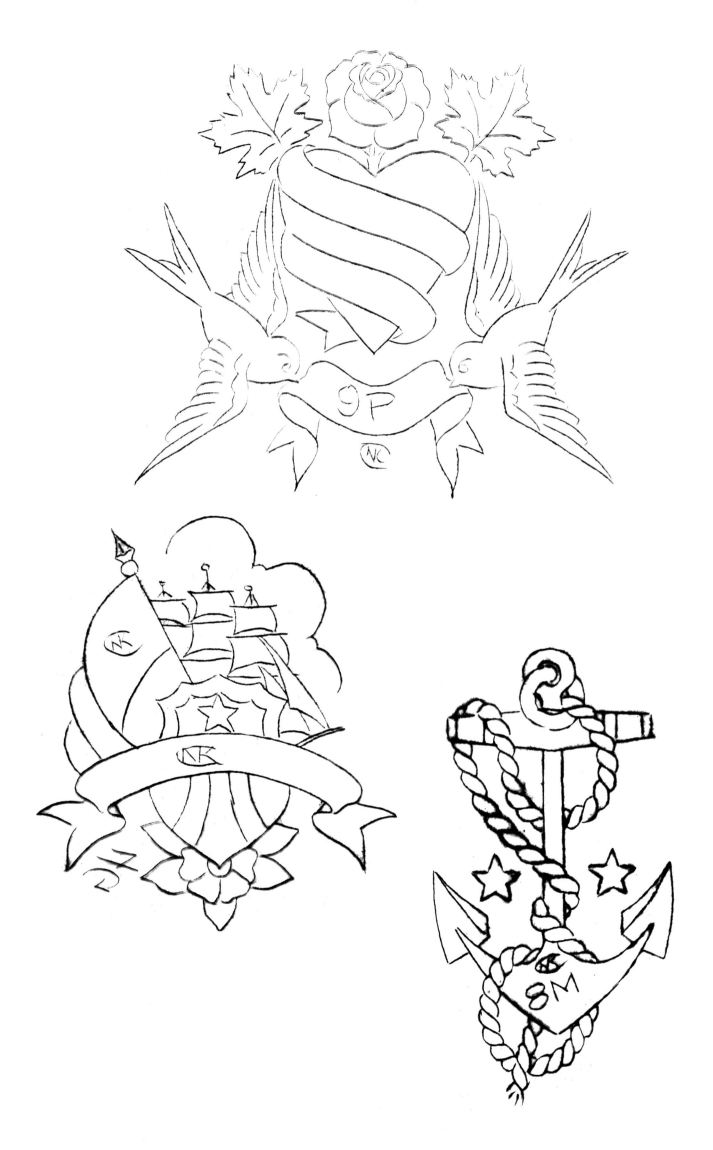

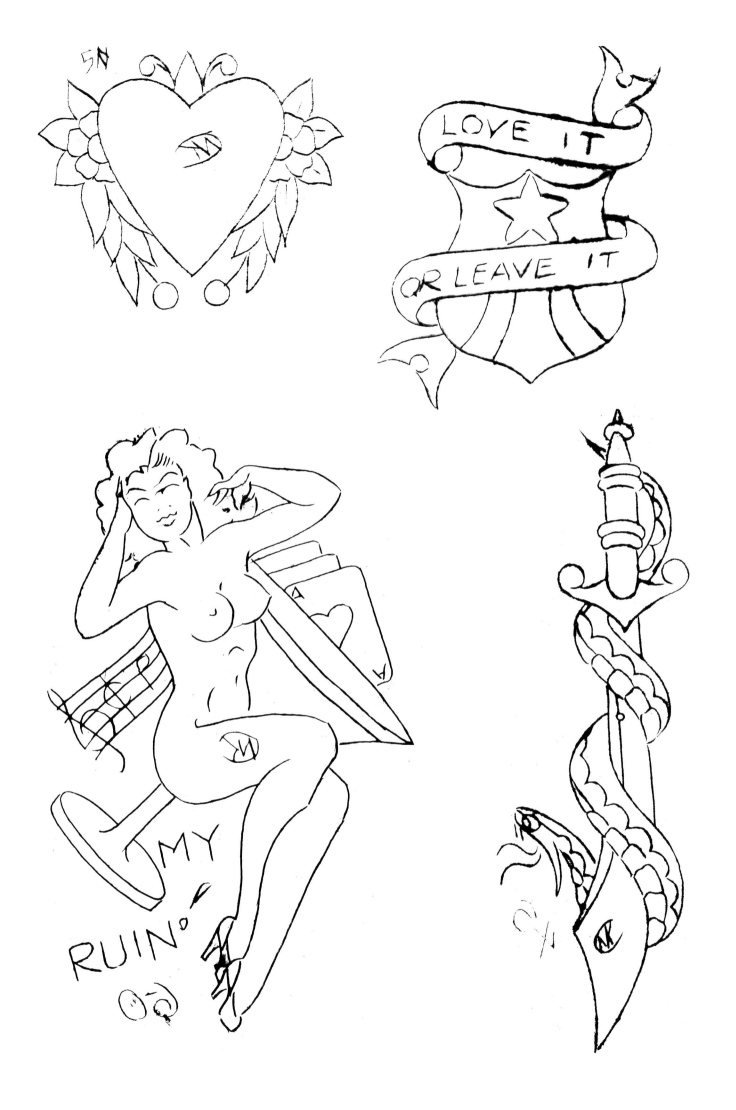

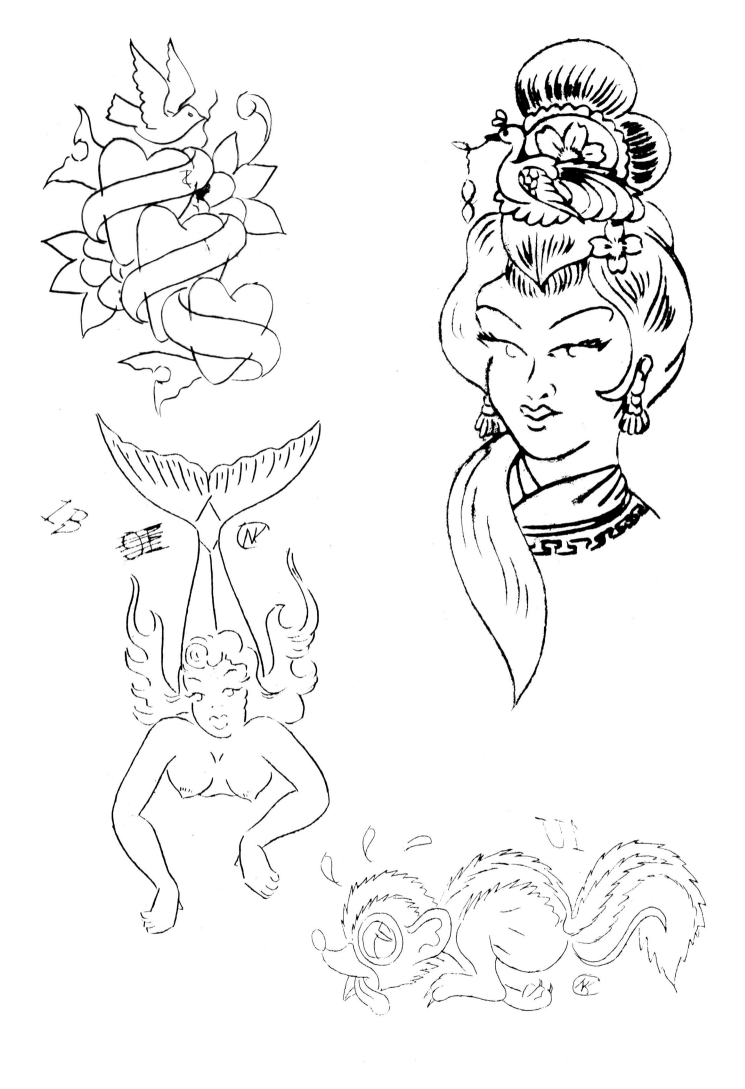

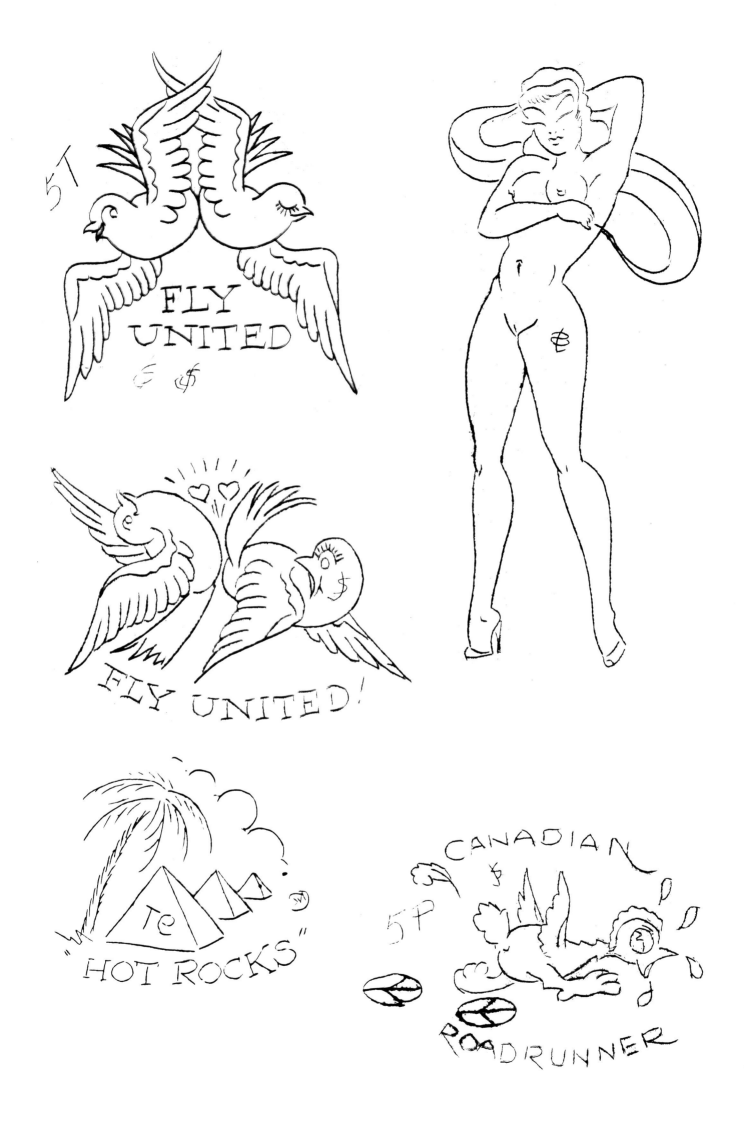

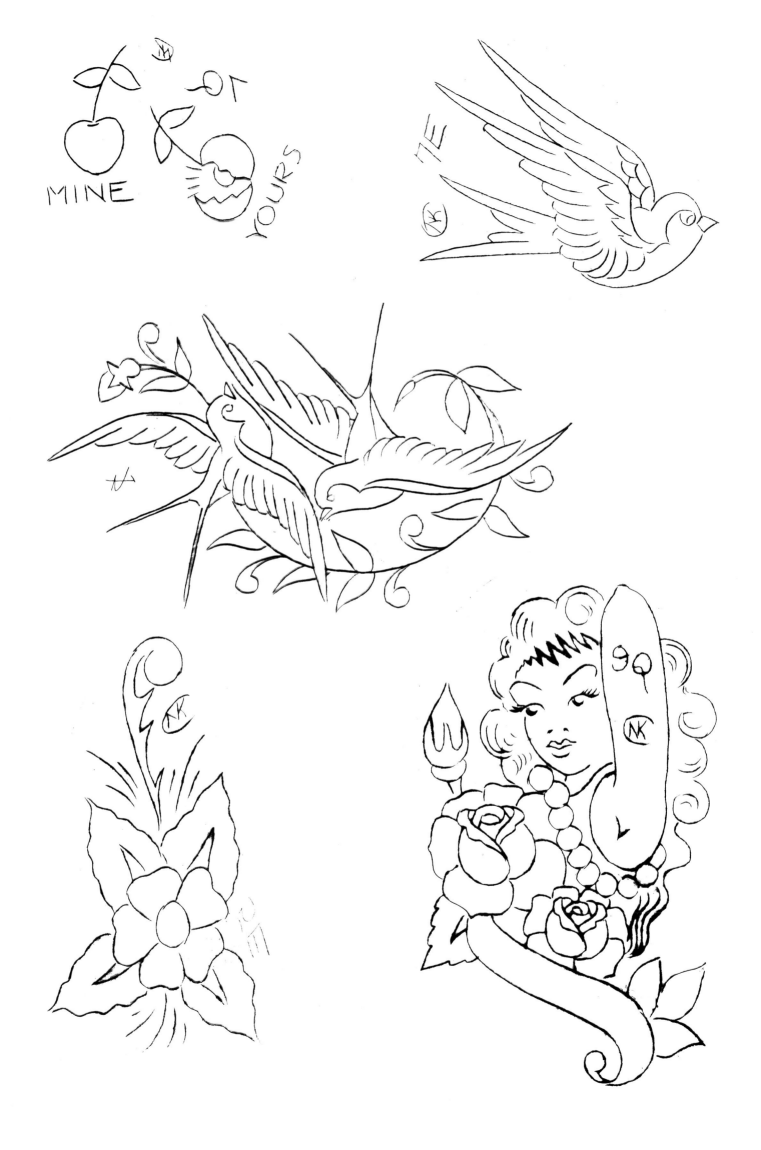

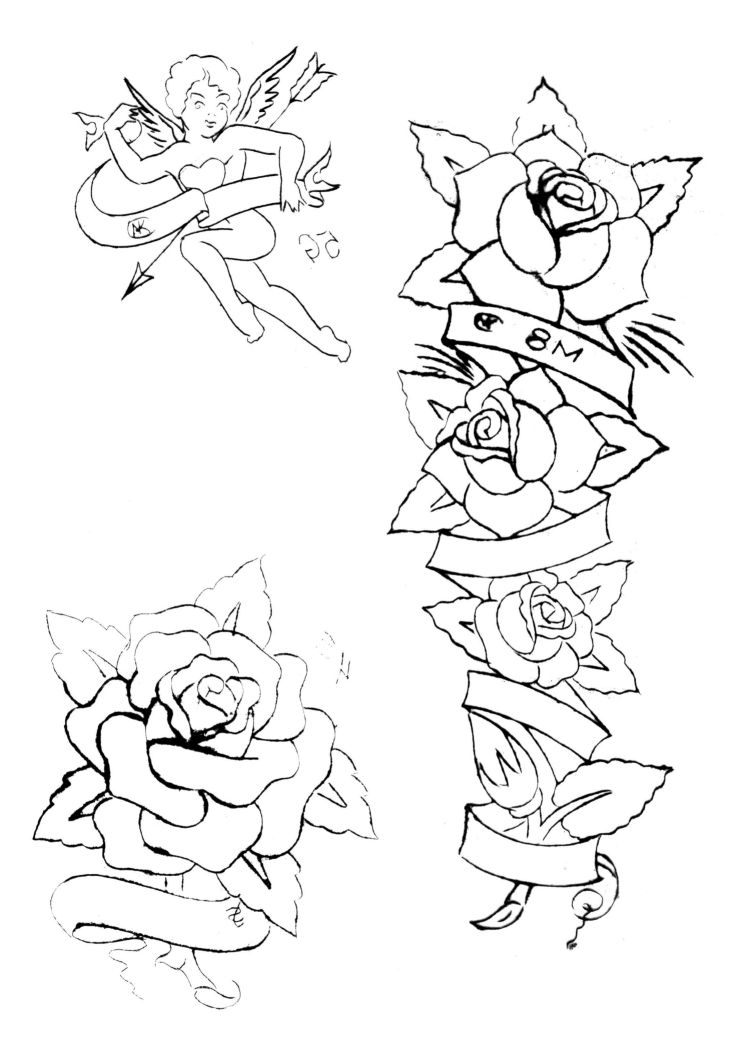

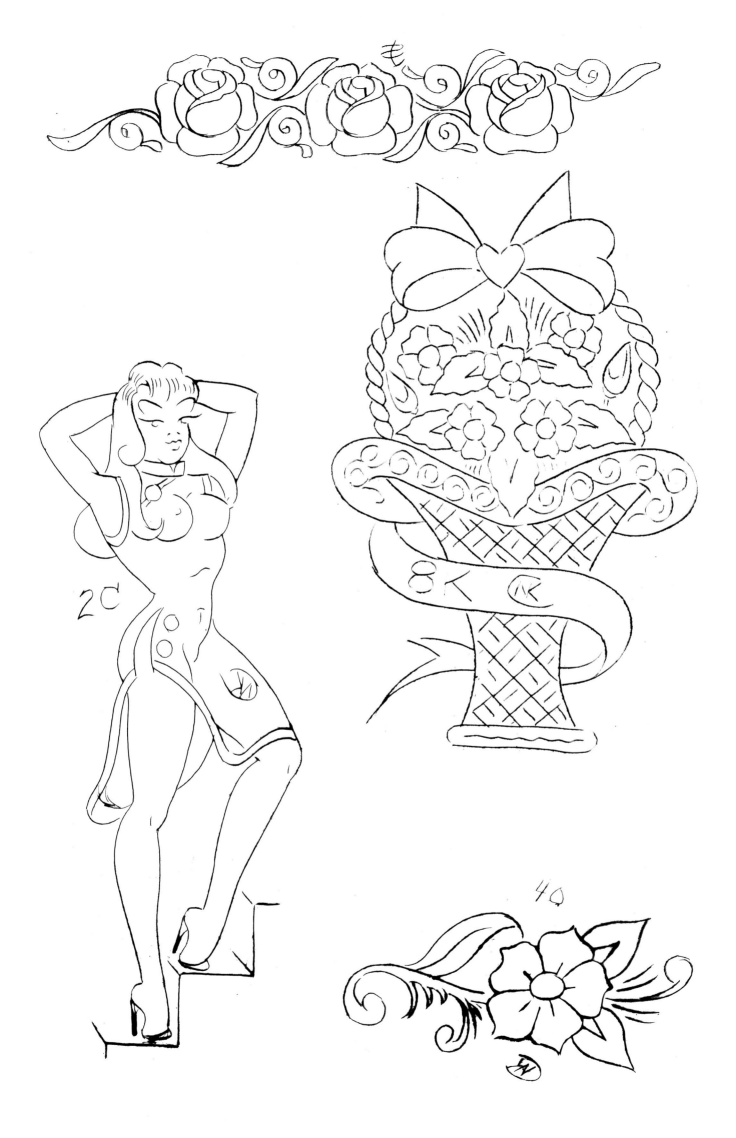

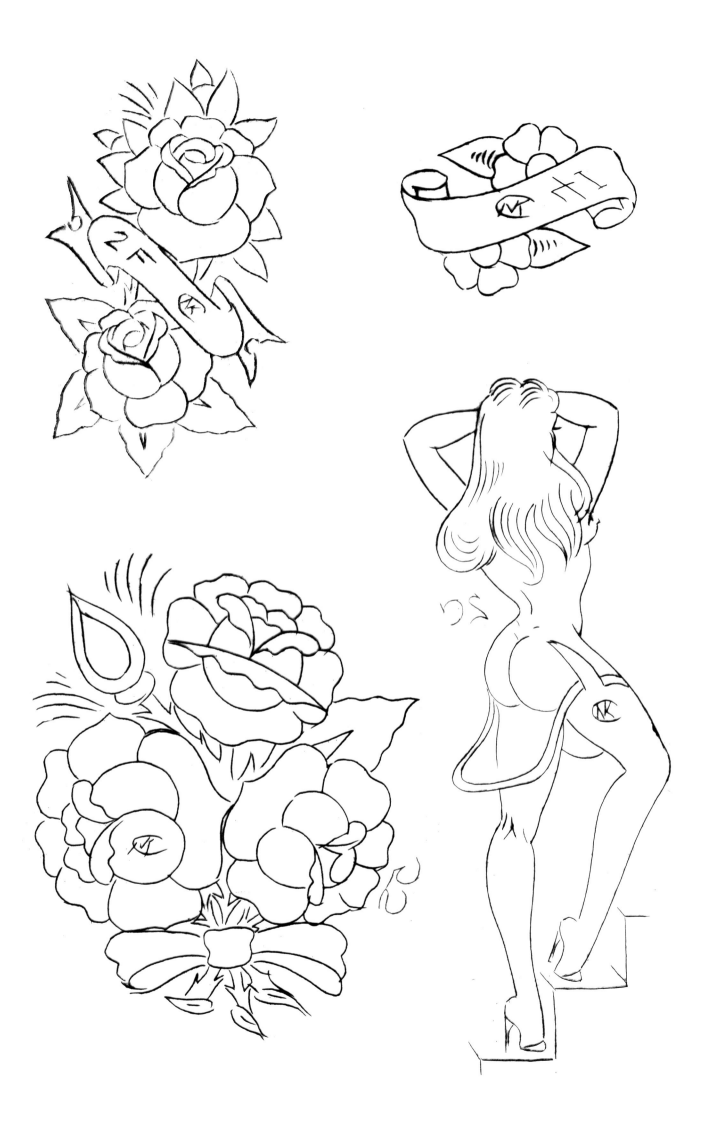

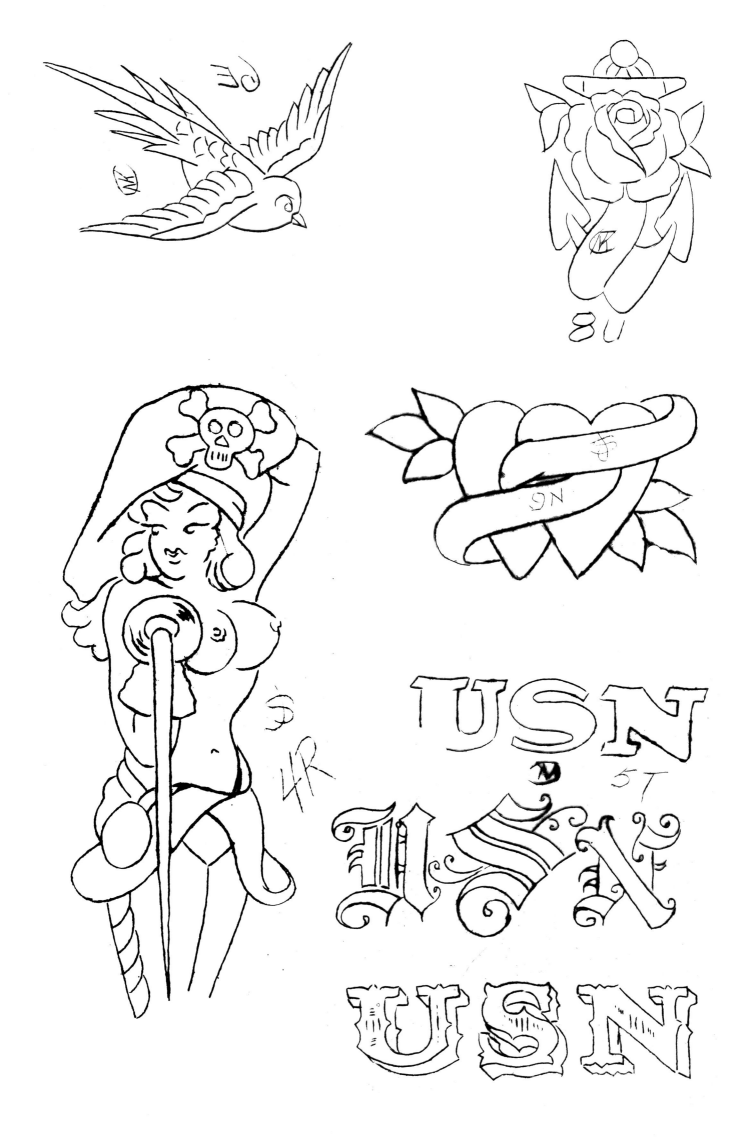

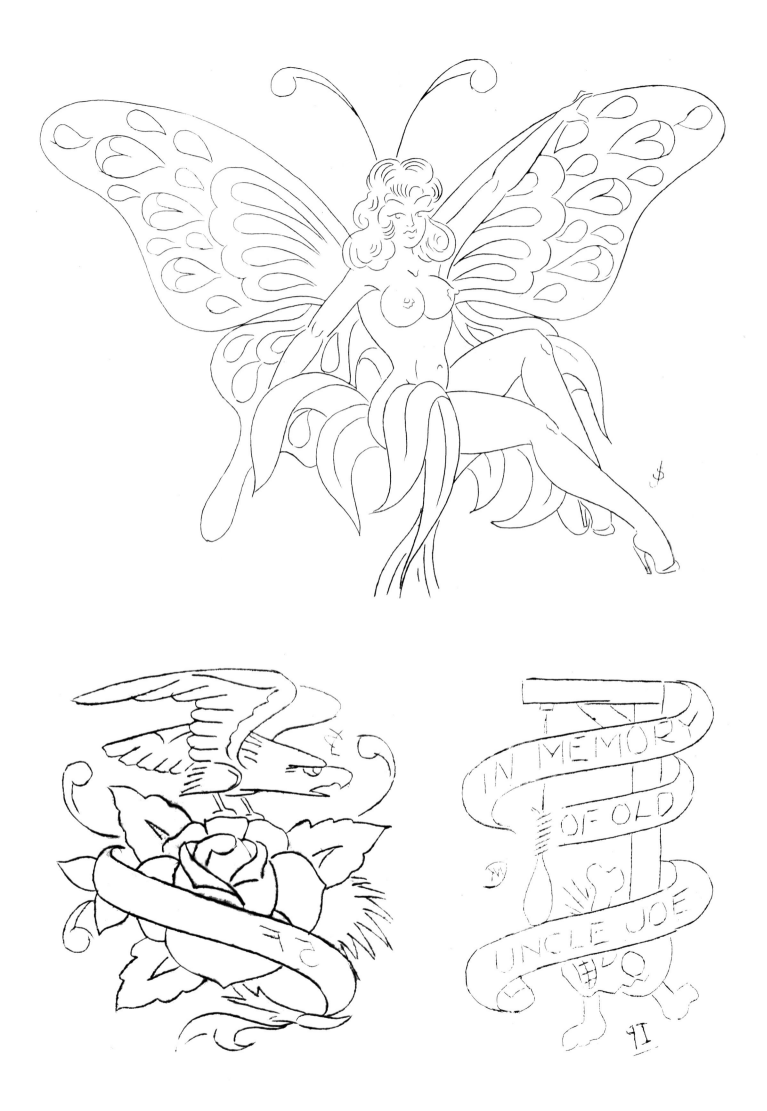

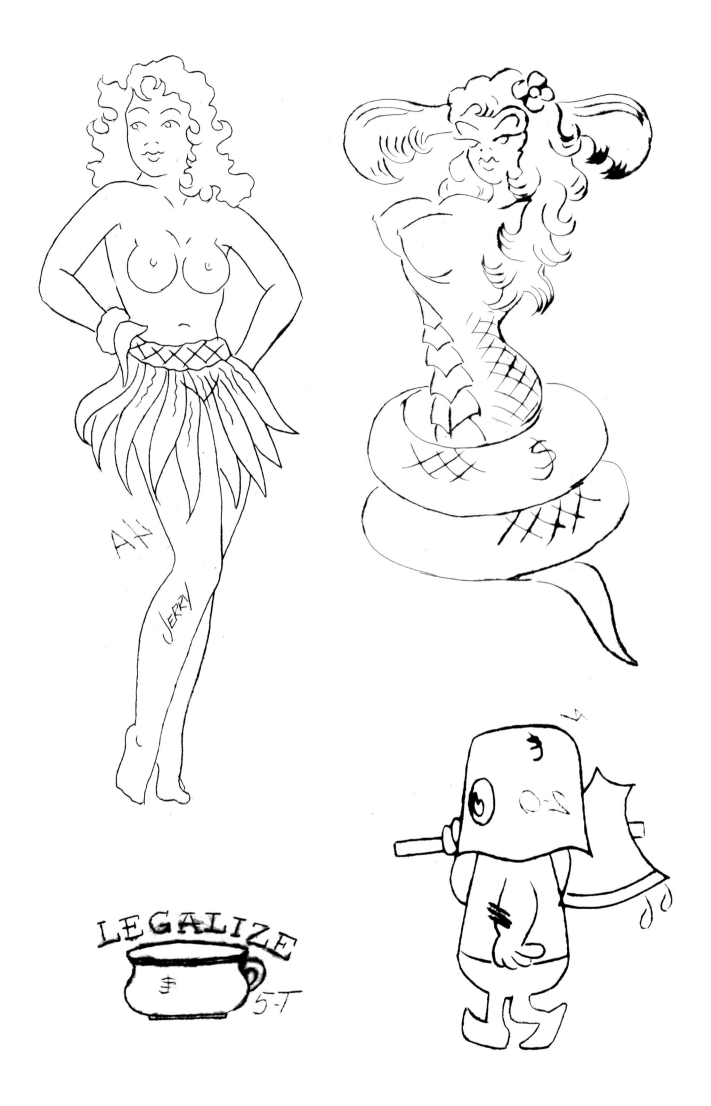

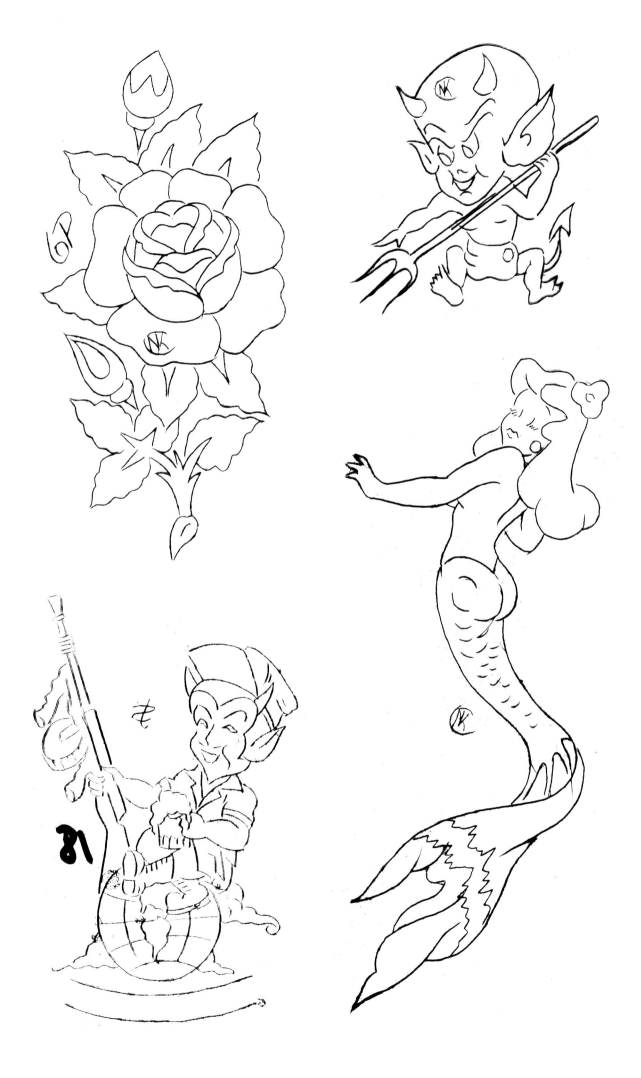

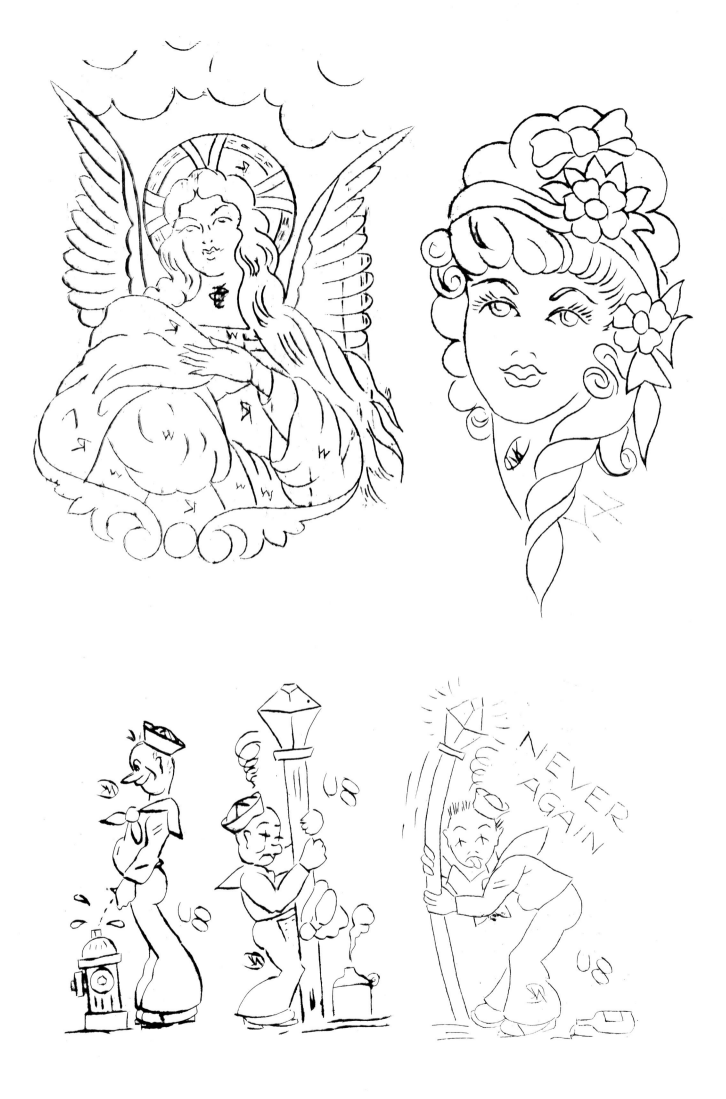

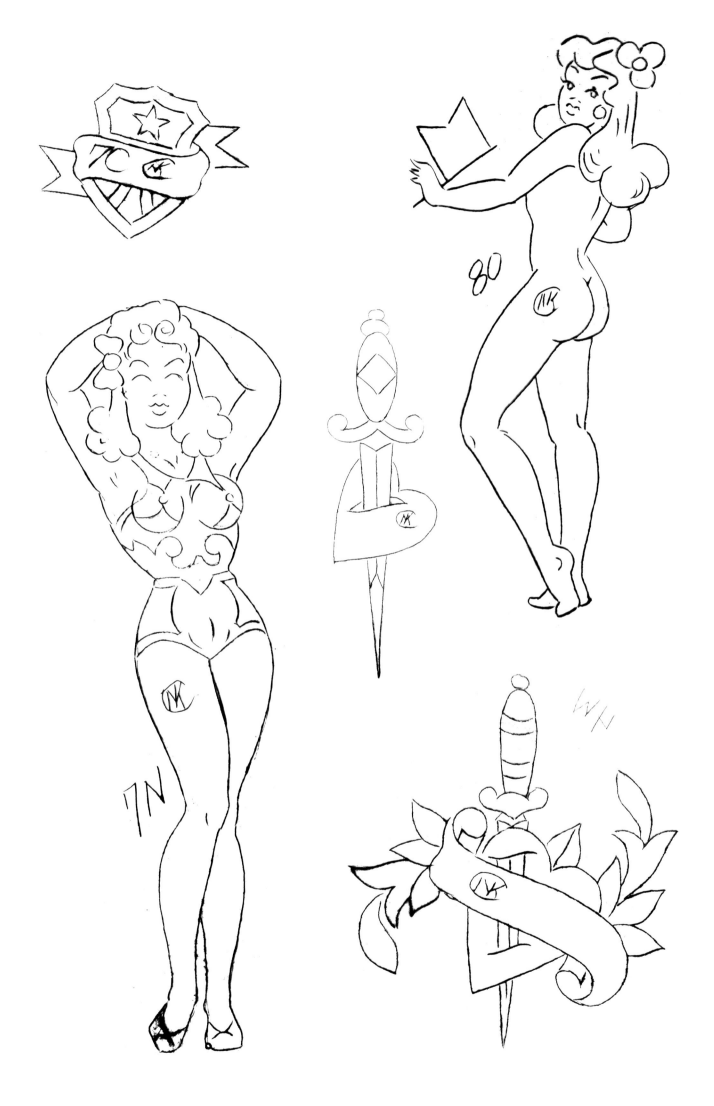

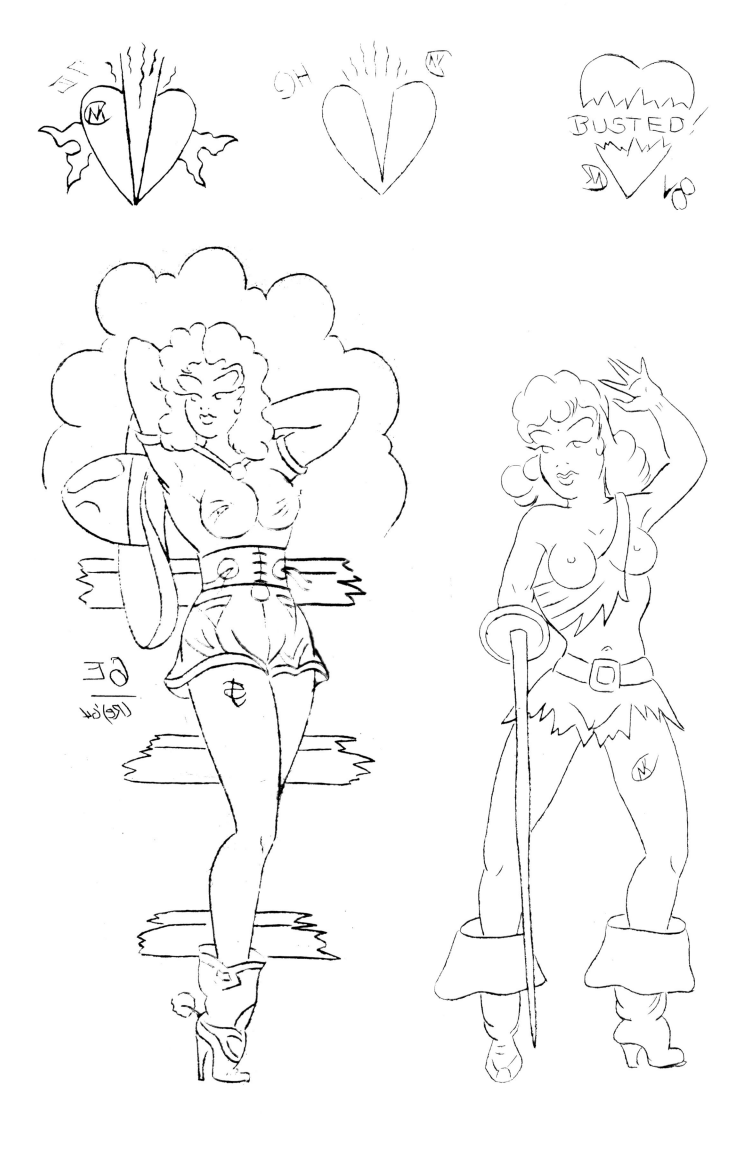

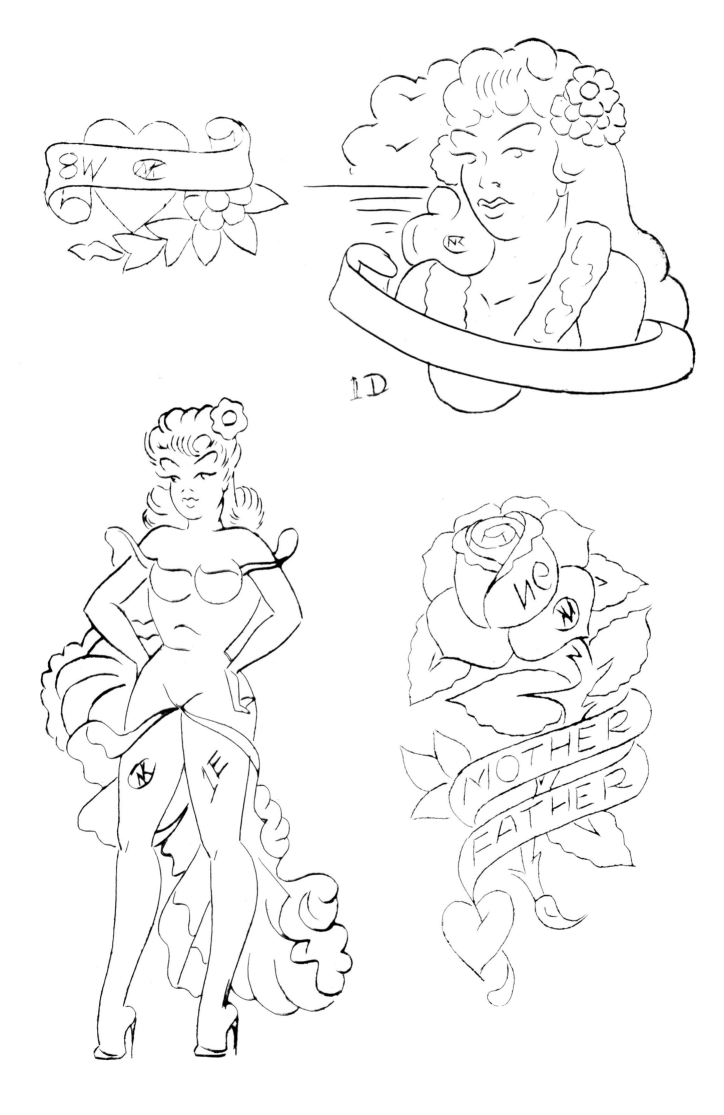

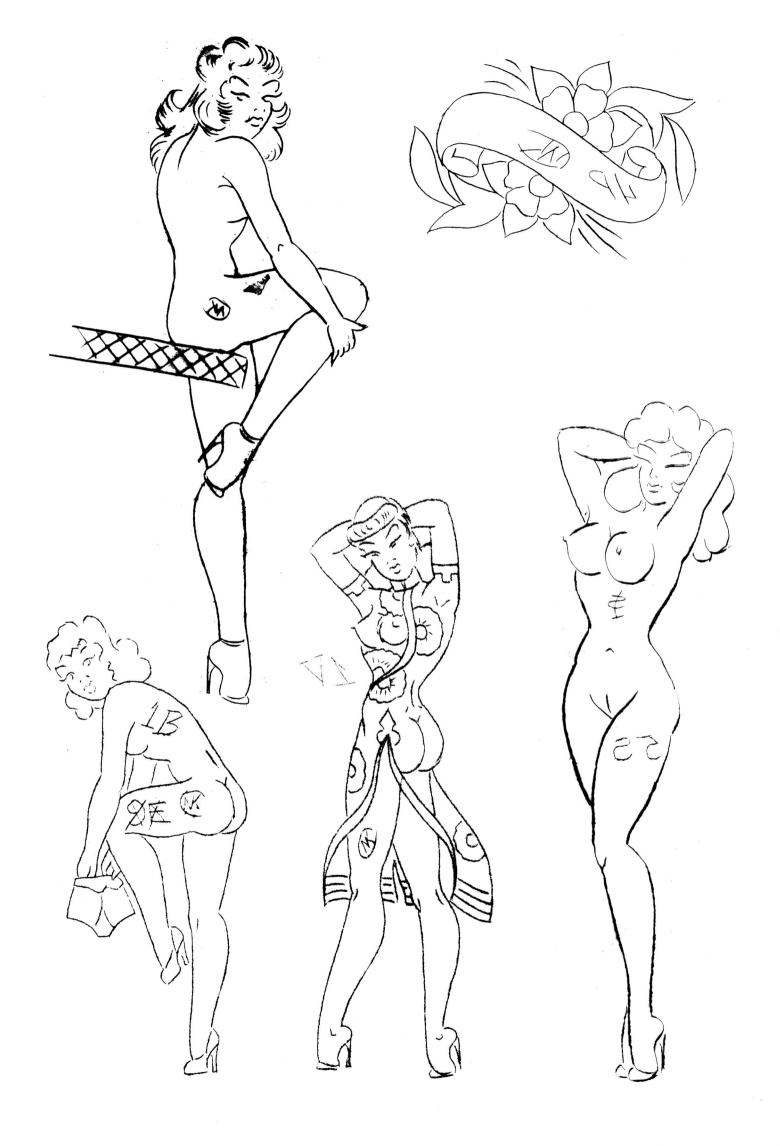

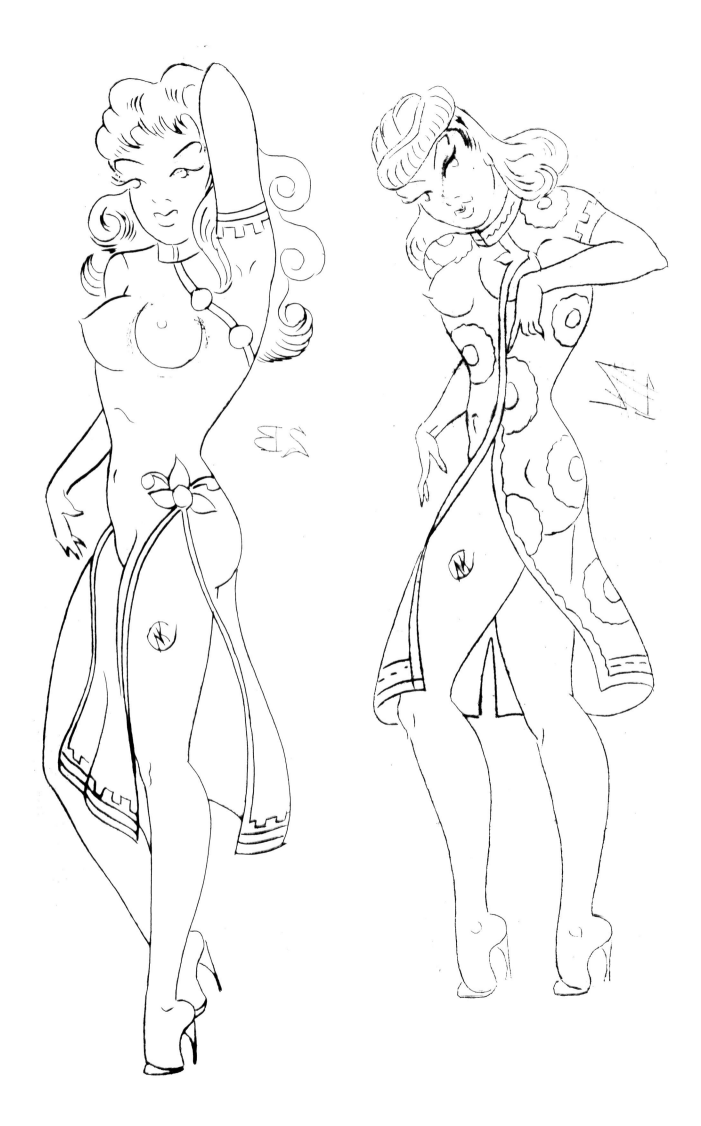

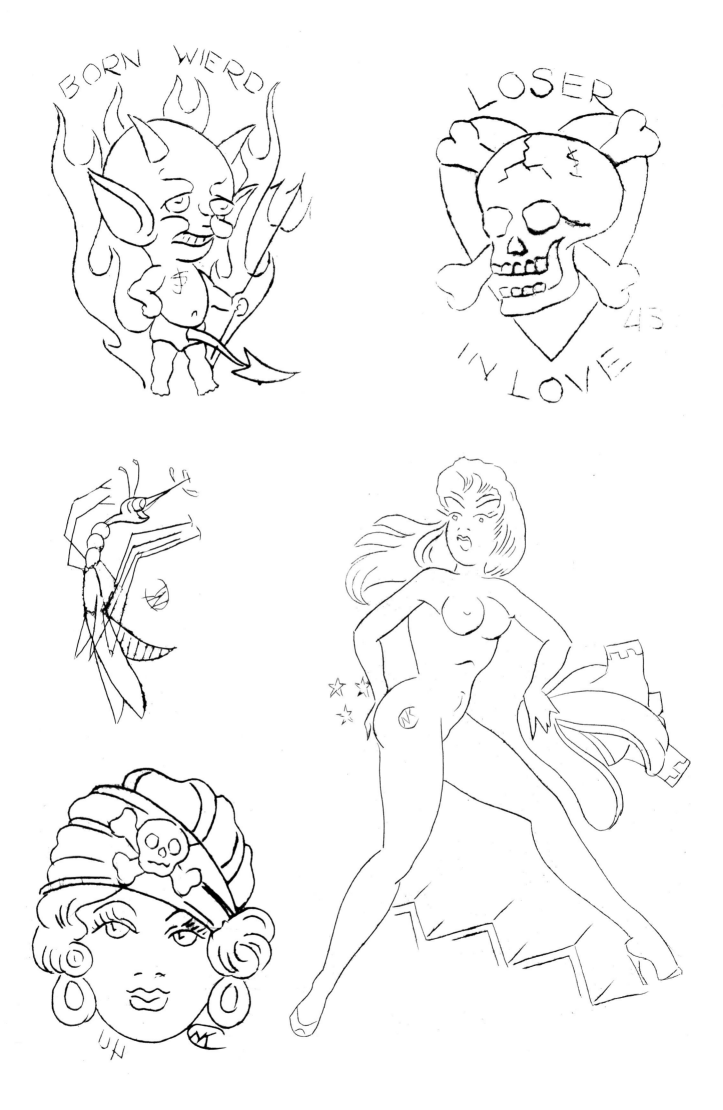

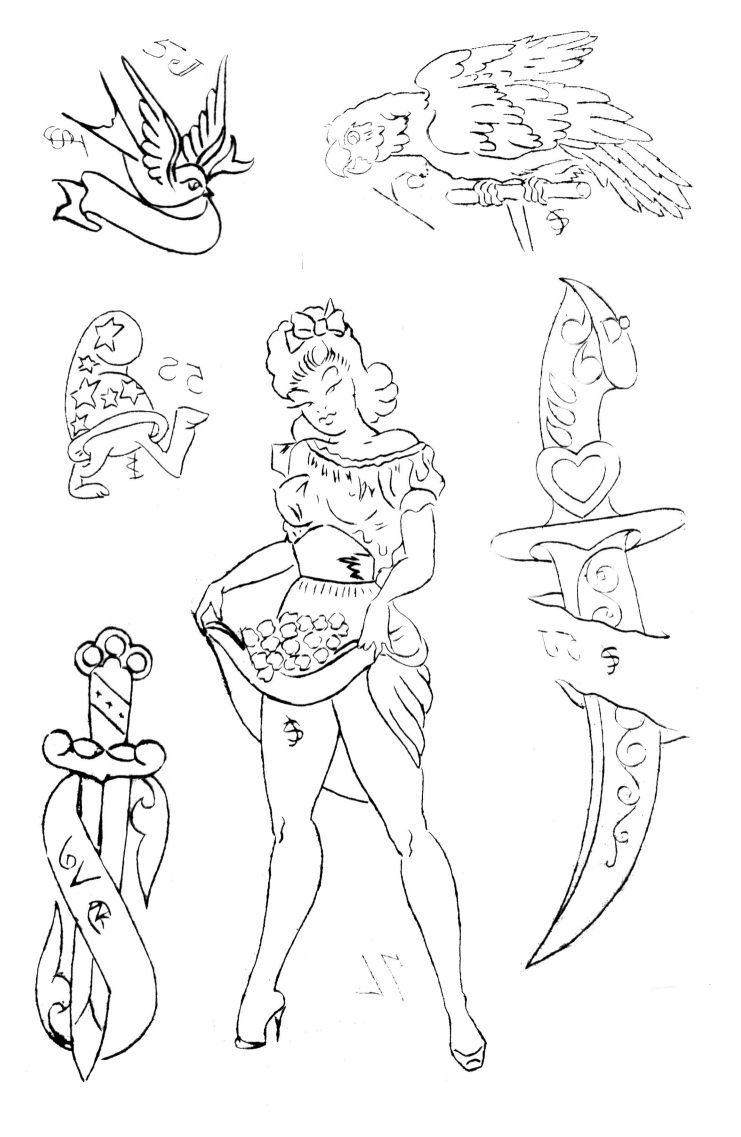

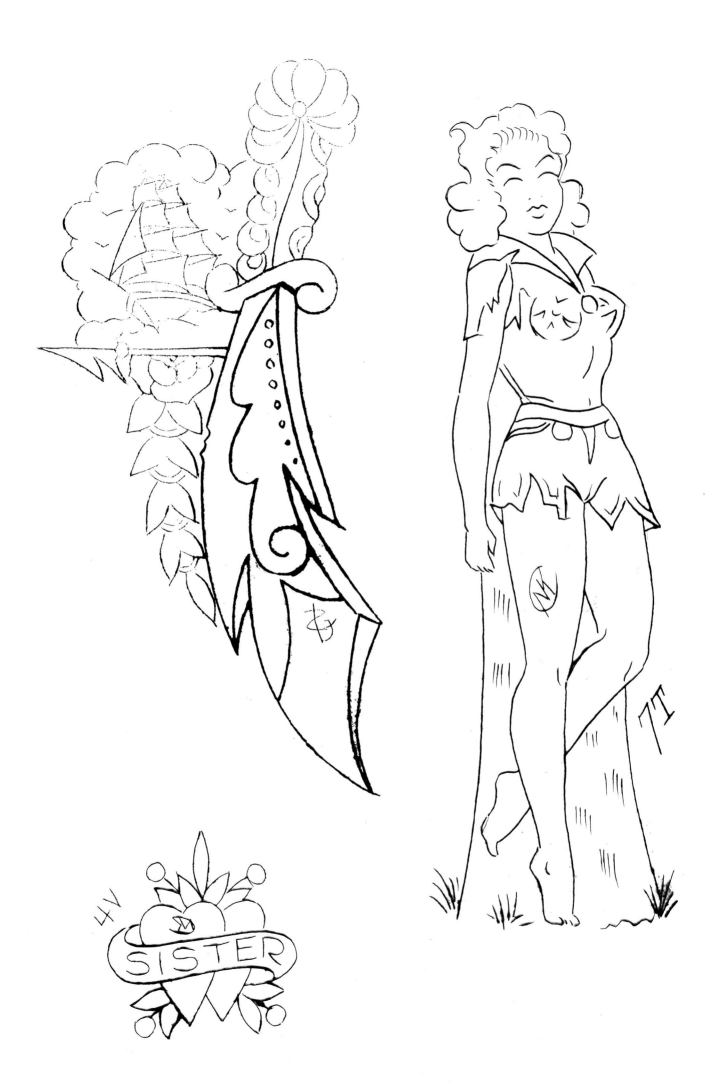

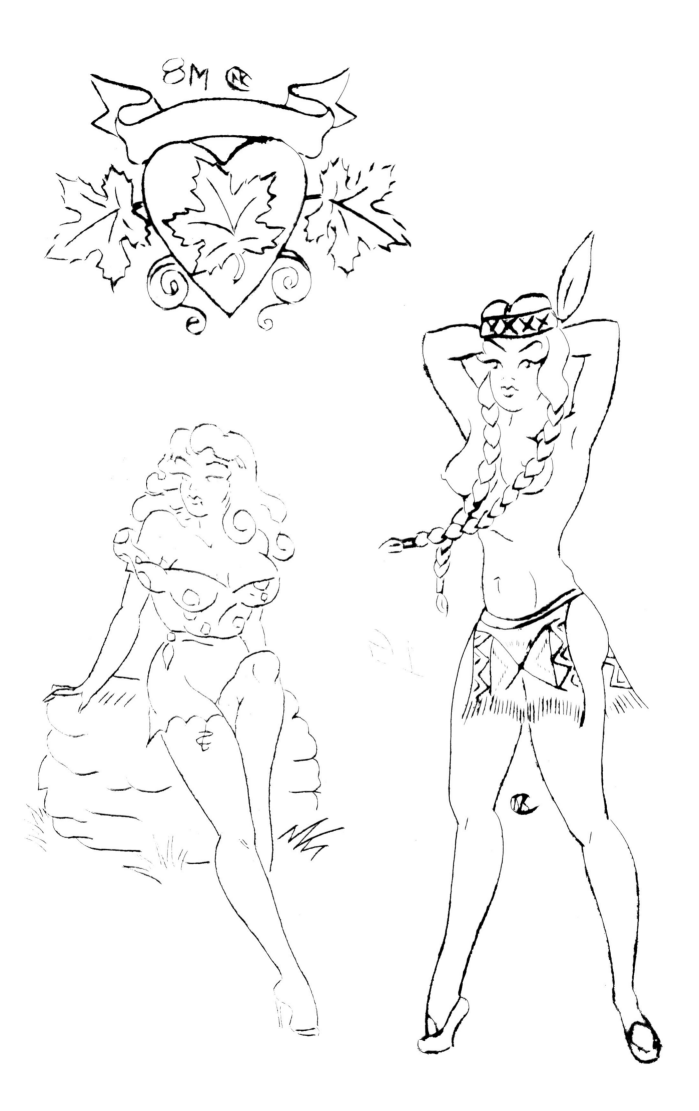

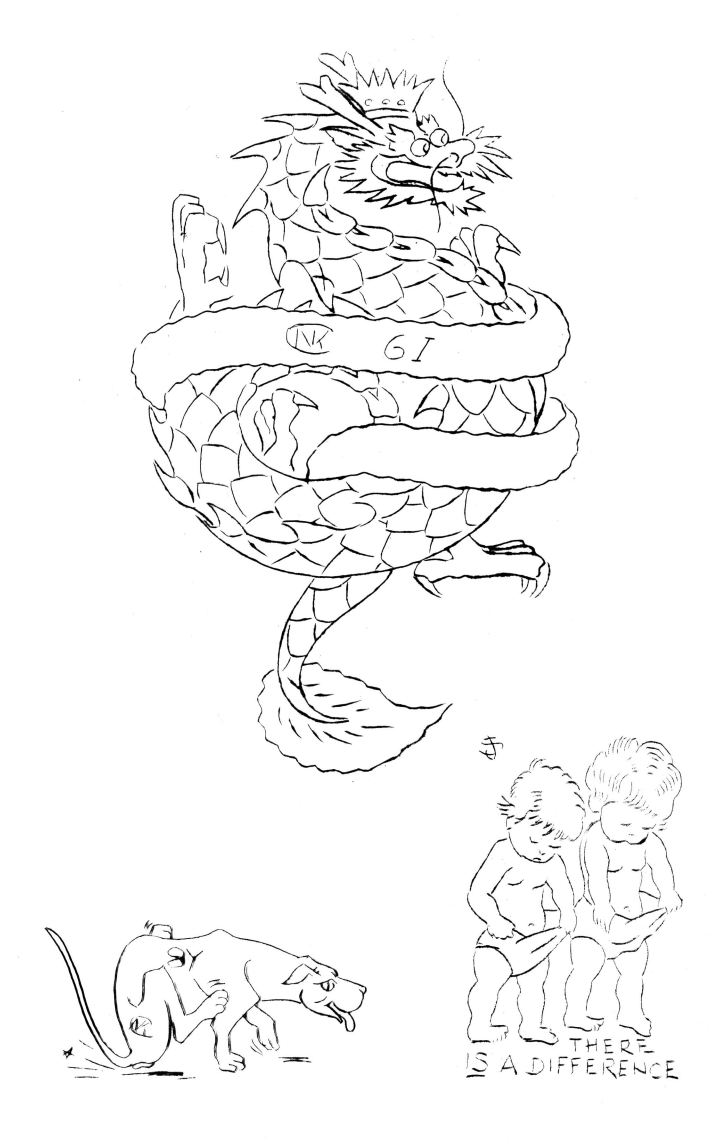

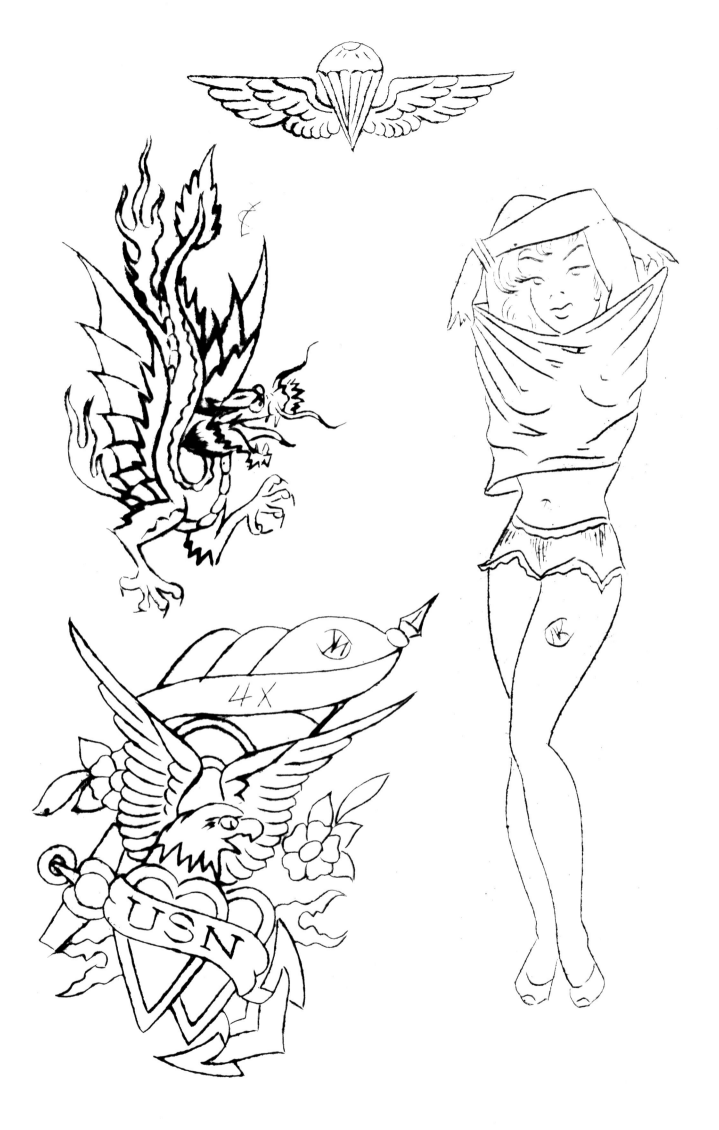

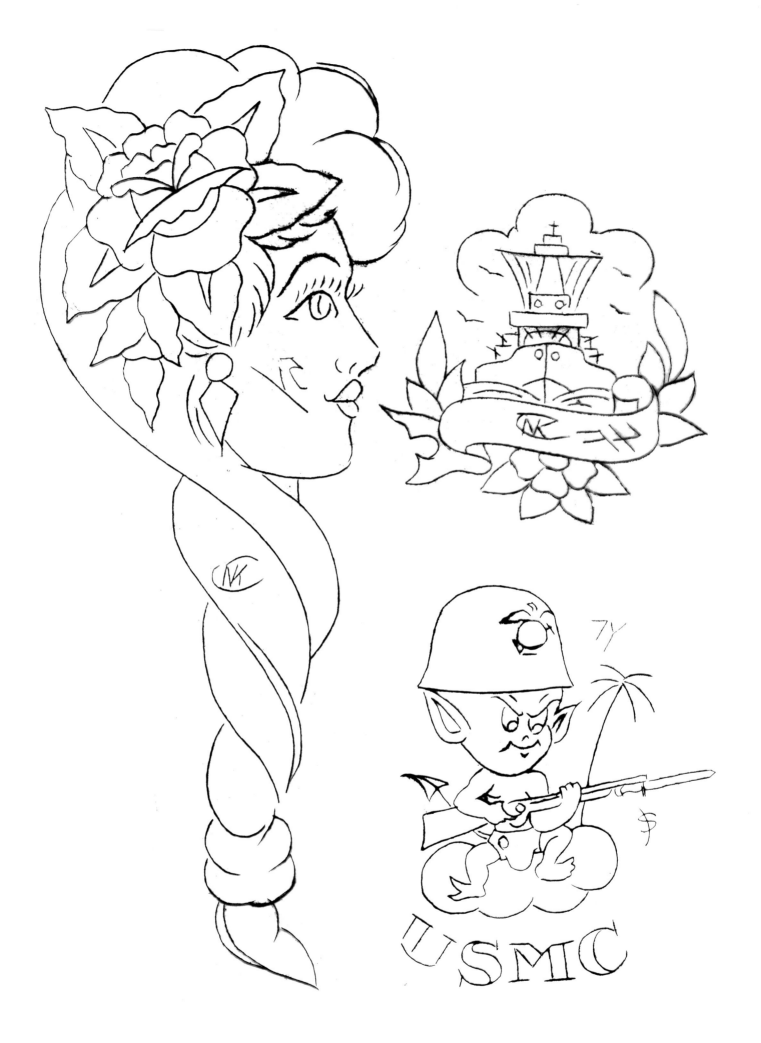

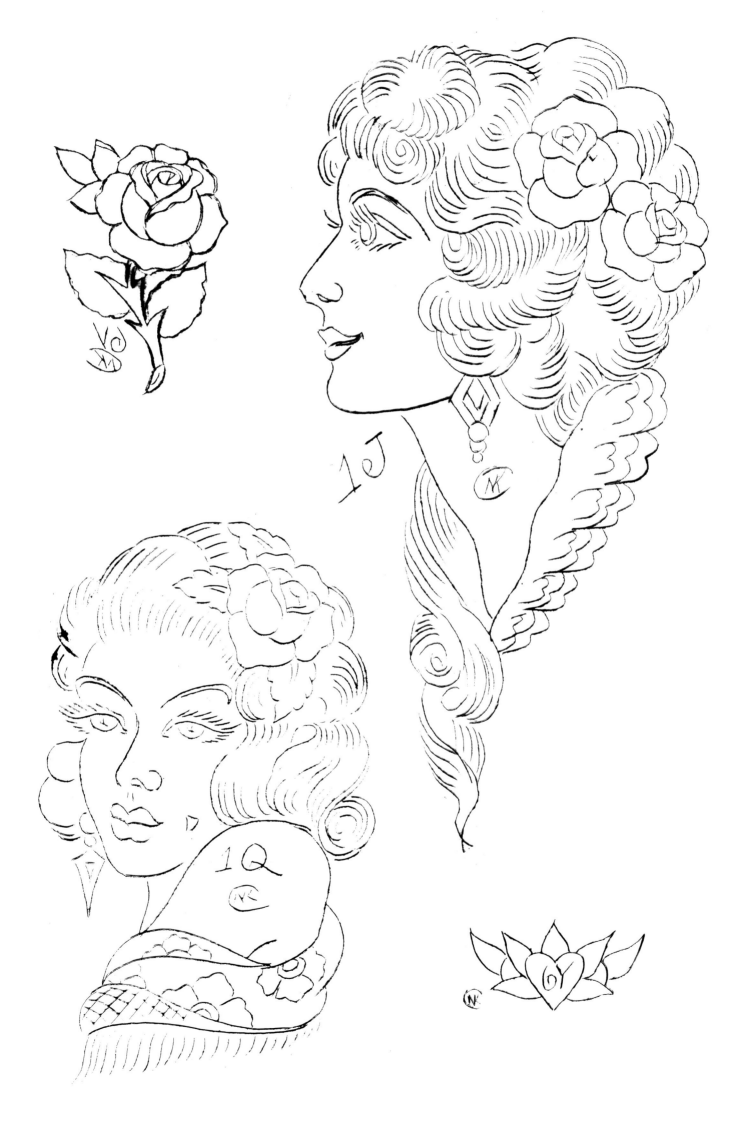

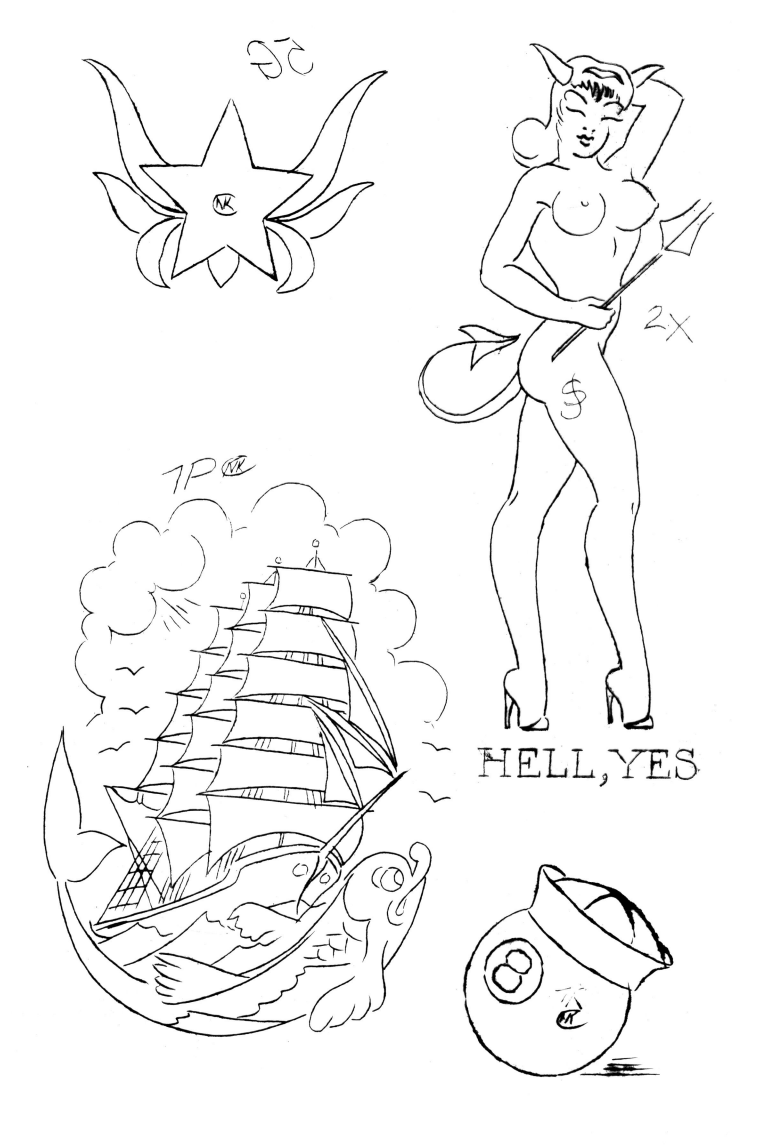

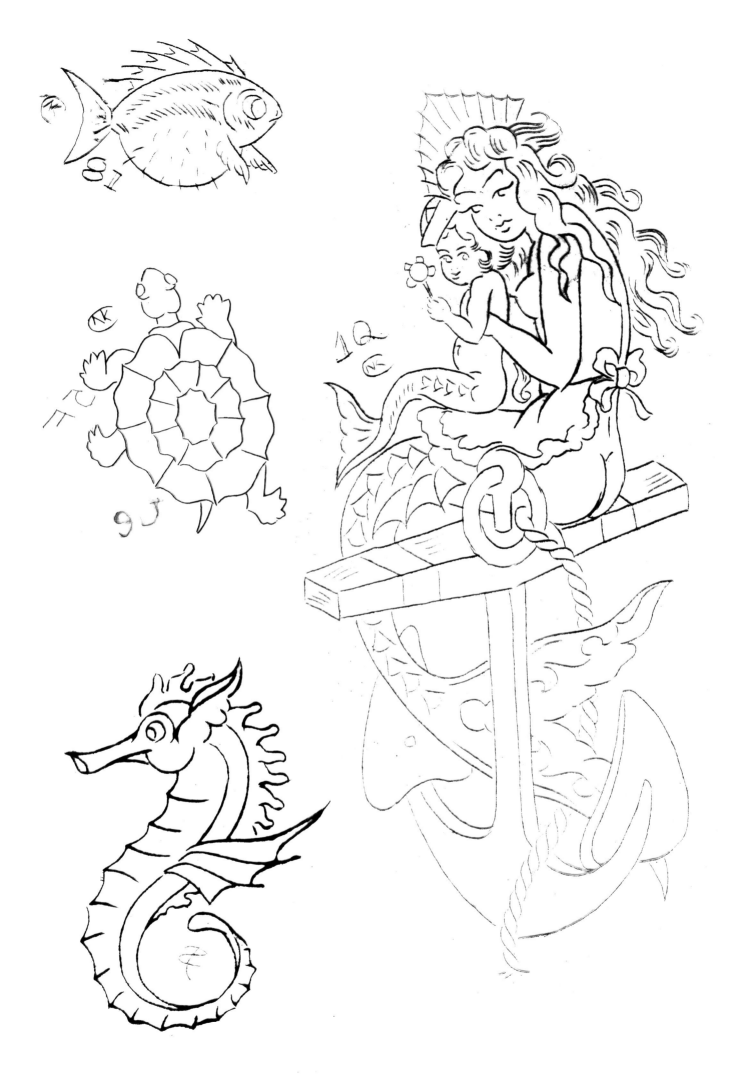

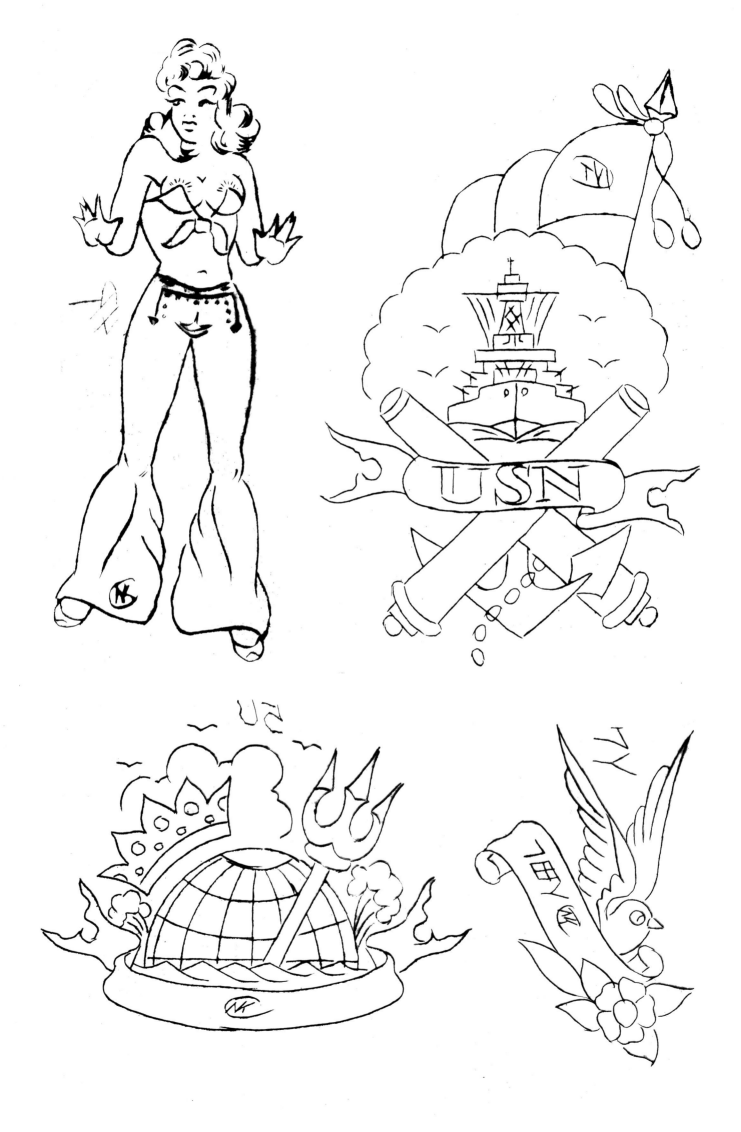

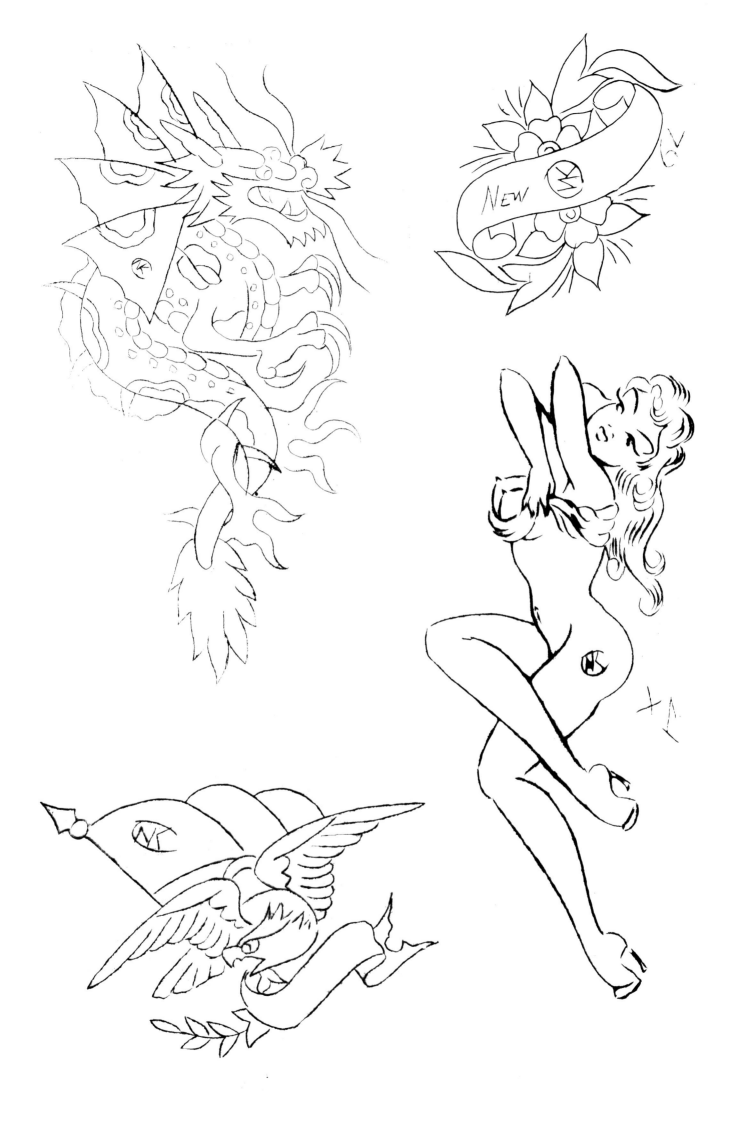

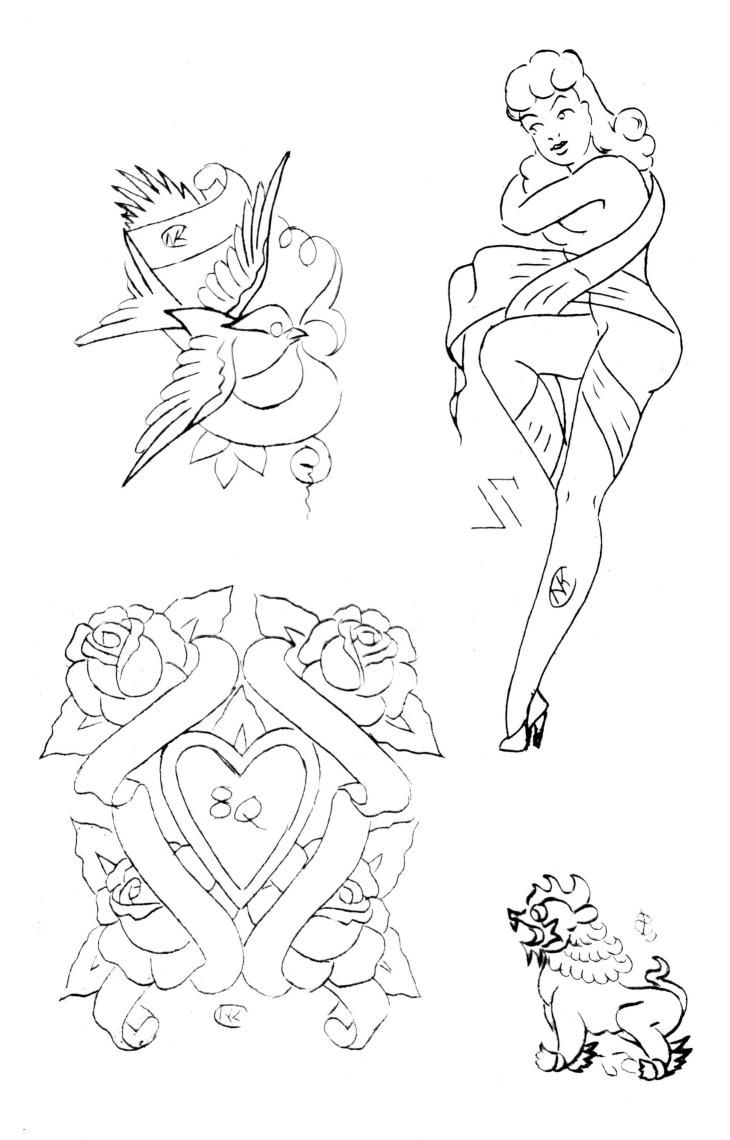

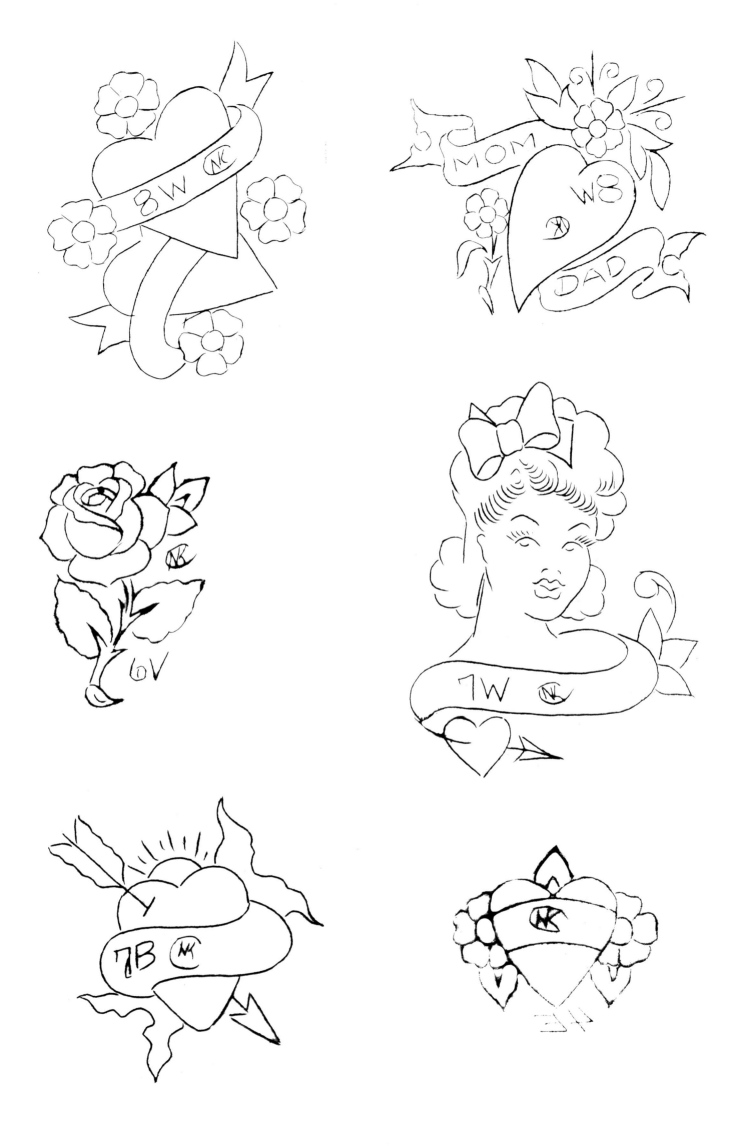

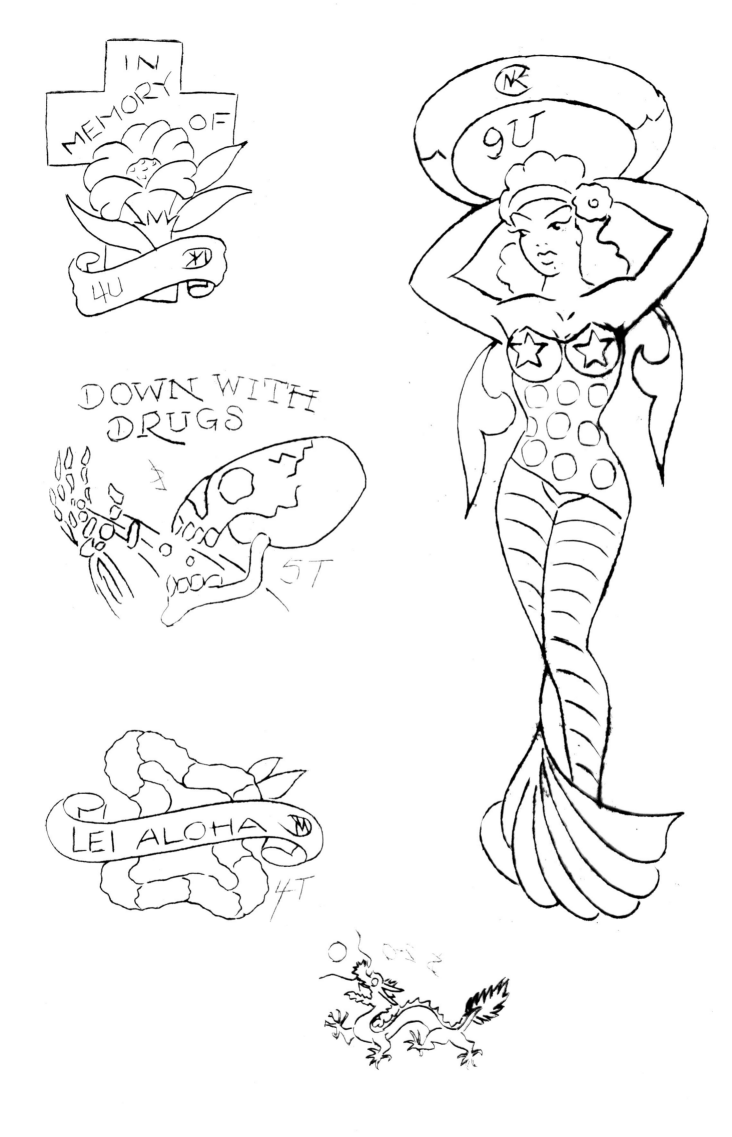

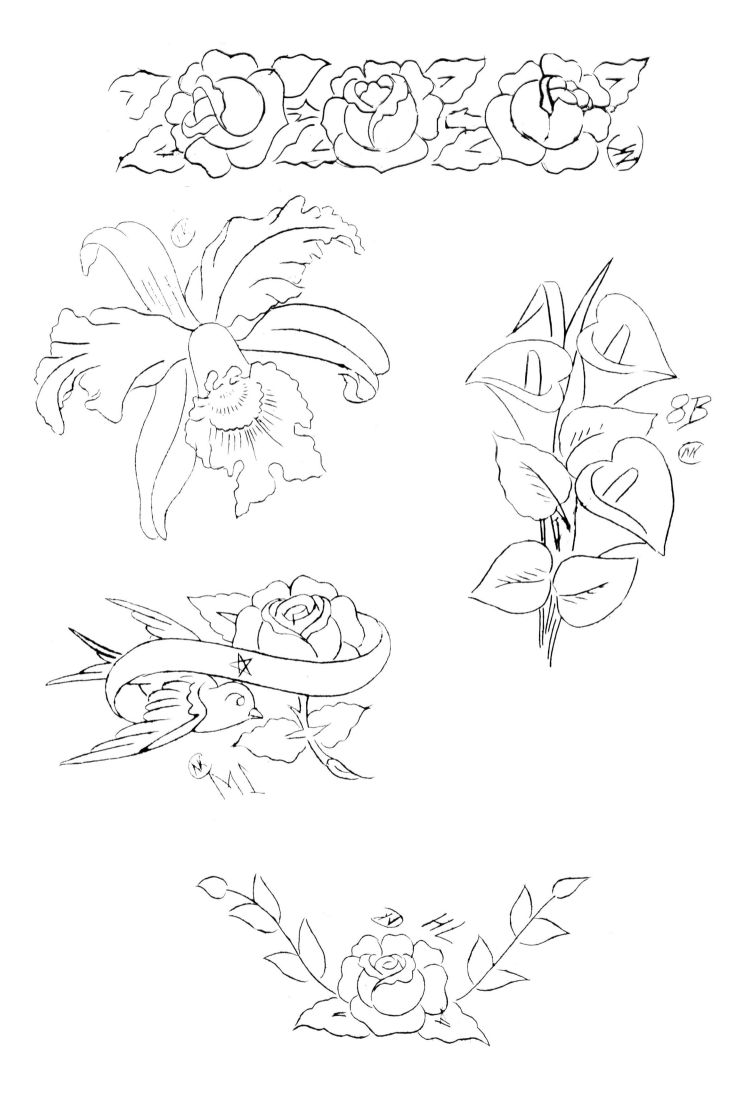

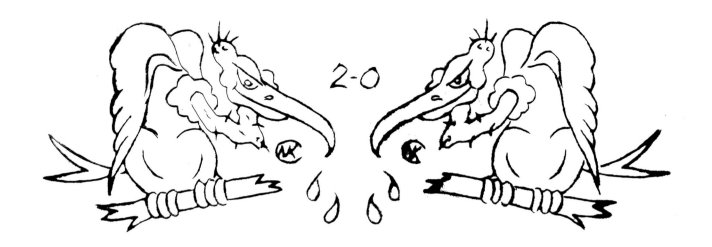

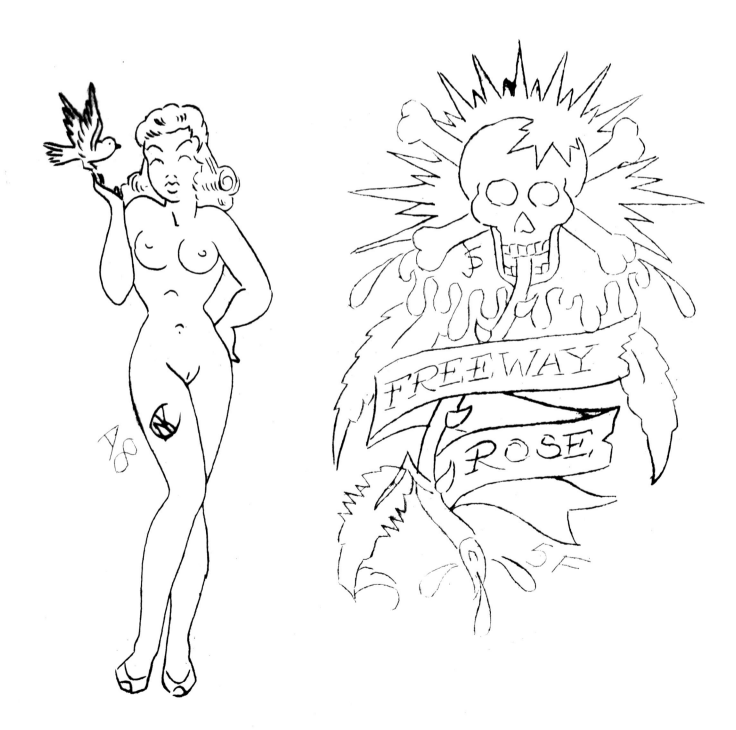

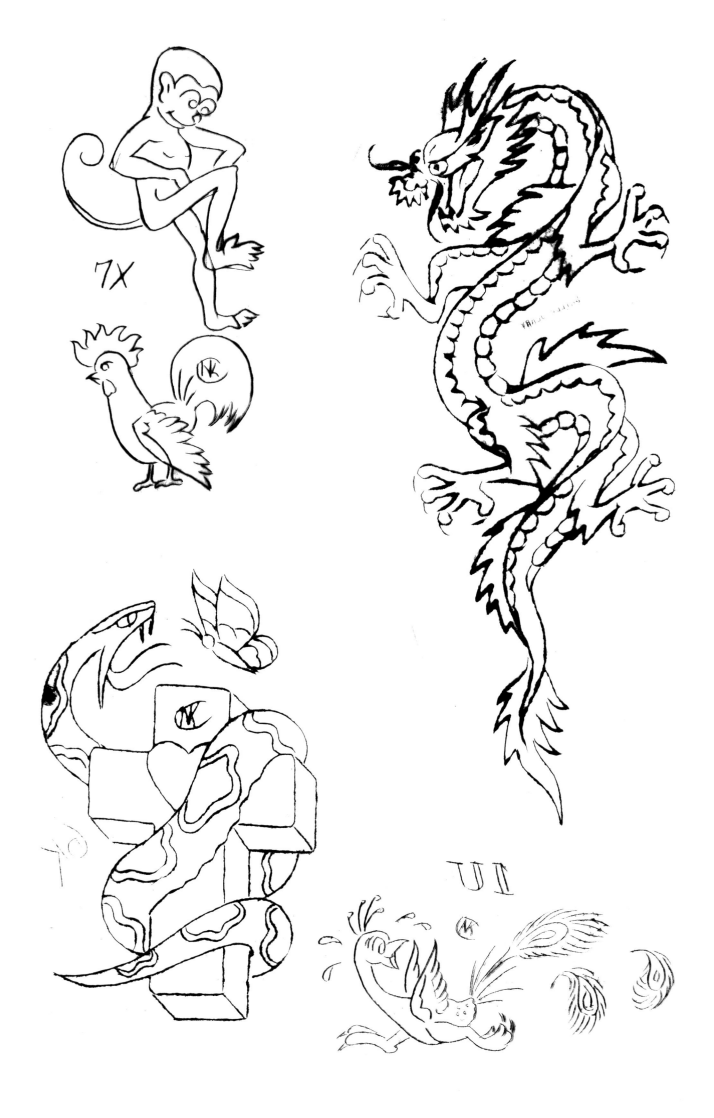

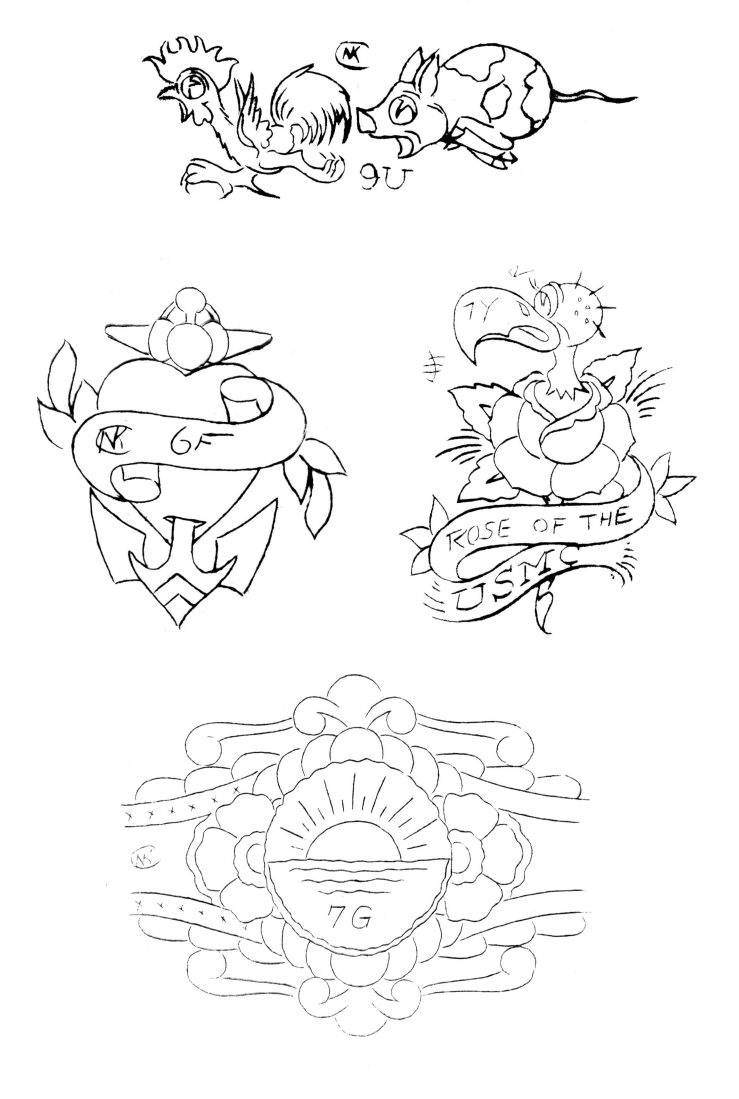

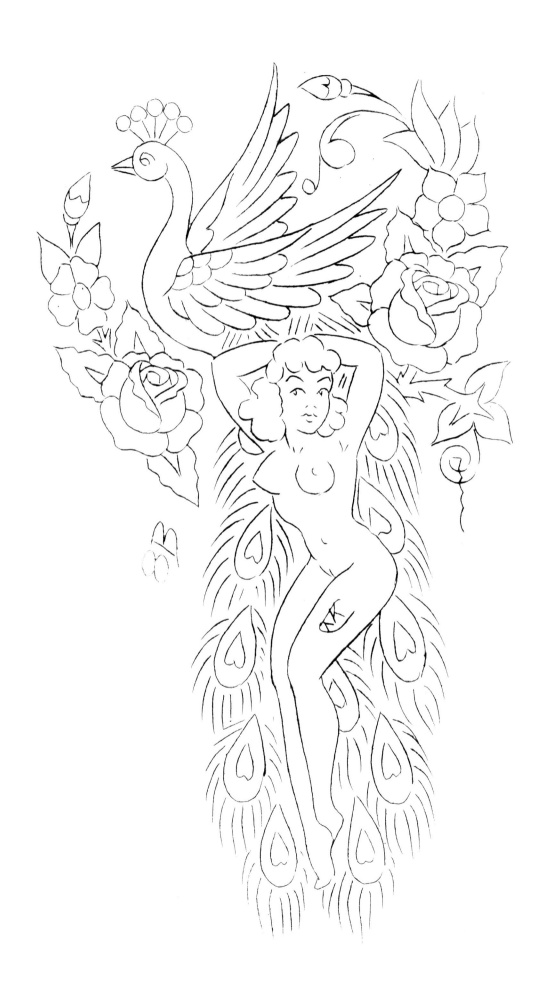

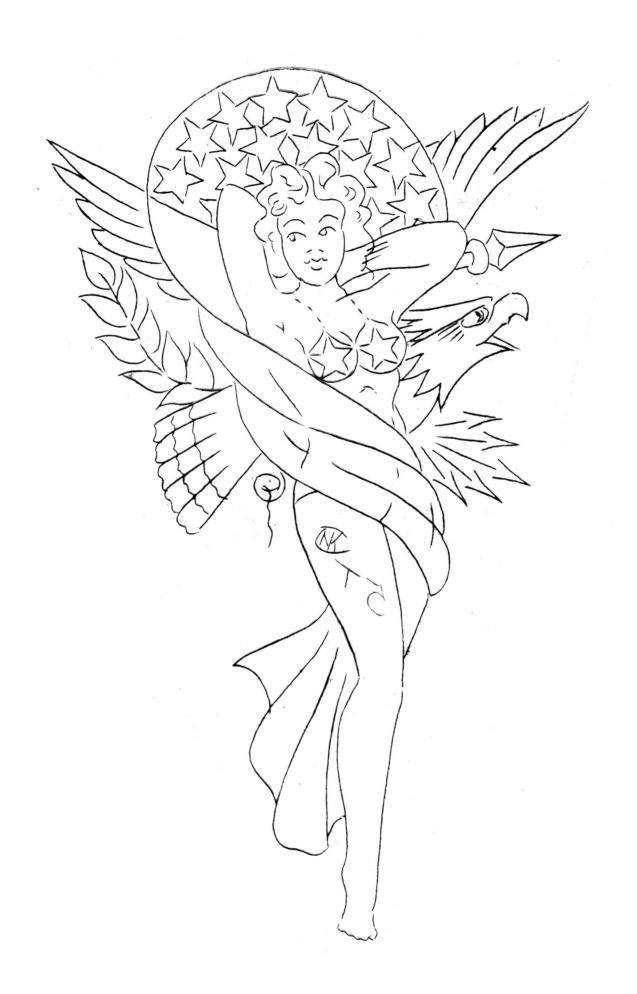

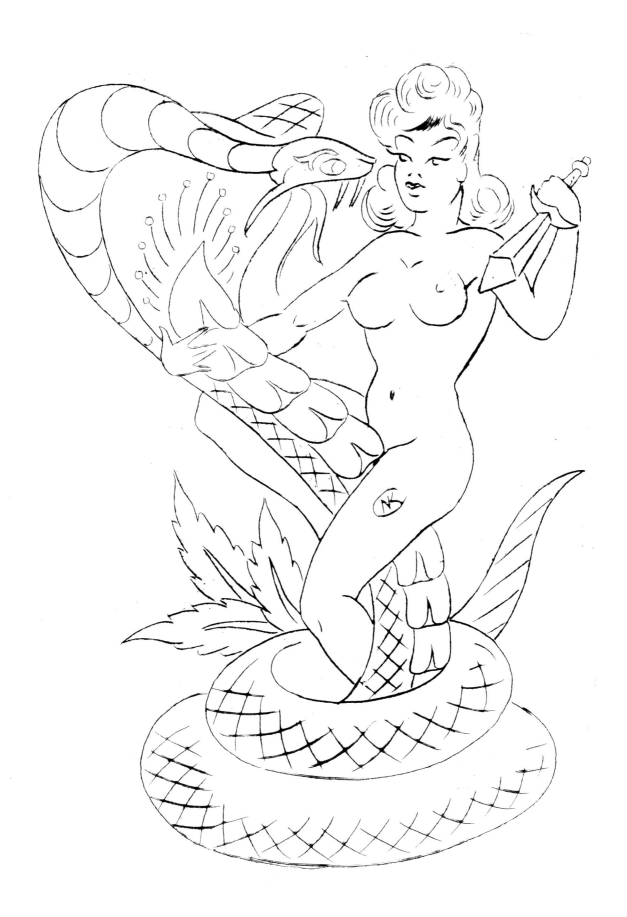

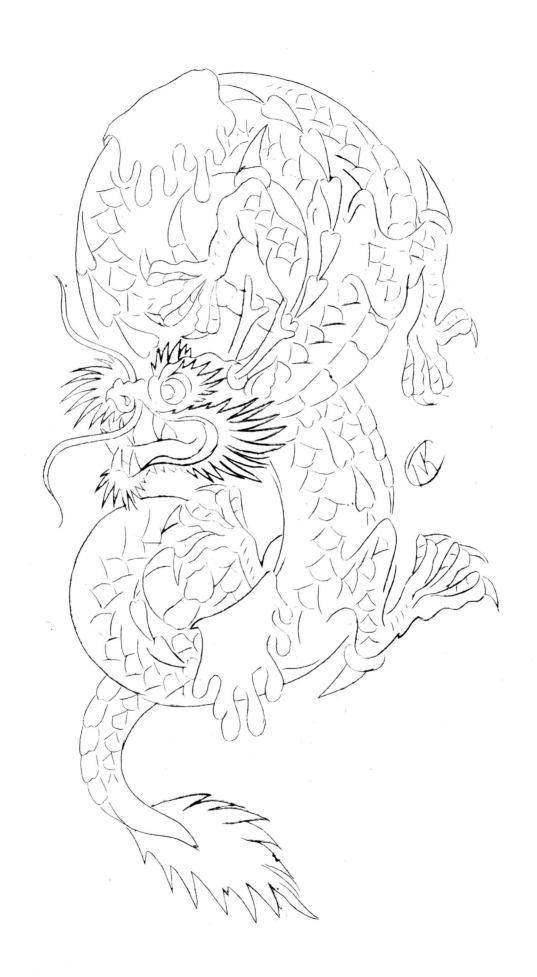

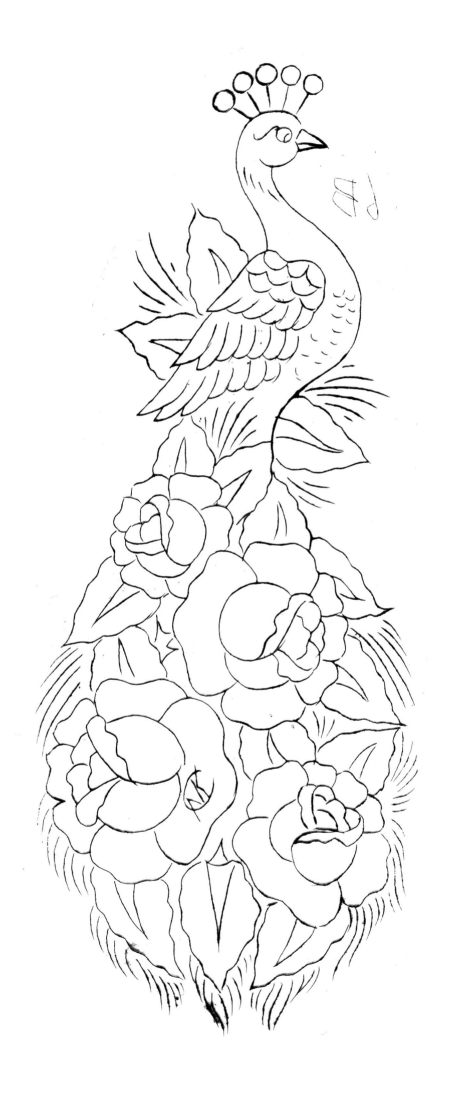

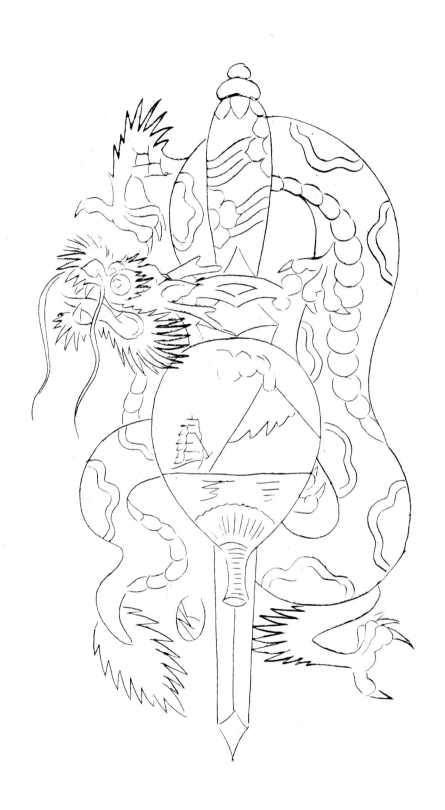